C+E

C000217692

# LOVING MEDICINE

Patients' Experiences of
the Bristol Cancer Help Centre

Rosy Thomson, BSc.MB.BCh

Foreword by Clive Wood, MSc.DPhil

Gateway Books, Bath

*First published in 1989*
*by GATEWAY BOOKS*
*The Hollies, Wellow,*
*Bath, BA2 8QJ*

*Set in 10½/12 pt Sabon*
*by Action Typesetting Ltd, Gloucester*
*Printed and bound by*
*Billings of Worcester*
*Cover design by Alan Peacock*

*British Library Cataloguing in Publication Data*
  *Thomson, Rosy, 1955*
  *Loving medicine : patients' experiences*
  *of the Bristol Cancer Help Centre*
  *1. Cancer patients. Care*
  *I. Title*
  *369.1' 96994*

*ISBN 0-946551-49-9*

# Contents

I would like to acknowledge most deeply and gratefully the love and support of Pat and Christopher Pilkington, Frank Rozelaar-Green, Yolande and Suzy Burgin, Cathy and Charlie Thomson, Kerry Davies, Ceinwen Cochrane, Penny Brohn, Jean Sayre-Adams, Jane Whistler, Geoff Bevins, Glin Bennett and Clive Wood; first and foremost for seeing me through fifteen years of medical training and latterly in encouraging and guiding me through my journey into Holism. Not only has this resulted in the creation of this book and many other exciting opportunities, but also in a profound deepening of myself and my practice of medicine. I am also greatly indebted to all of the patients and their families, doctors and therapists who so willingly and openly shared their innermost thoughts and feelings with me thereby making this book possible. I would also like to thank Tim Gayton for rescuing me from word processor madness, Dr Michael Wetzler for his excellent contribution to the book and Alick Bartholomew for his great vote of confidence in publishing it.

This book is dedicated to all of you with my very fondest love.

# Foreword

This book is about transformation. It describes a process through which ordinary people reach depths of understanding and acceptance of themselves and their lives that most of us never achieve. It is the supreme irony that they do so after having been diagnosed as cancer sufferers. It is the supreme affirmation that they do so after being patients at the Cancer Help Centre. The Cancer Help Centre is celebrating the end of its first decade. Rosy Thomson's book represents a series of snapshots of people who have passed through the Centre during those ten years. She produced it by the simplest and most direct methods — by talking to them and letting them talk for themselves. What they say shines through these pages. It is a testament to Dr Thomson's belief that "the state of a person's energy has far reaching consequences both for their own health and for the health of those around them". The Bristol philosophy is very much about that exchange and the interchange of energies between the patients and the staff, a process which has powerful influences on them both.

But is this really healing? Sceptics will point out that no alternative cancer therapy has yet been shown to prolong any patient's life-span. And as Rosy Thomson herself insists, the vignettes in this book represent only a tiny handful of the thousands of patients who have passed through Bristol. Maybe she could have produced a similar collection of much bleaker cases. The answer, as Professor Joad might have said, depends on what you mean by healing. If the sole criterion for any treatment is an increase in longevity, then the Bristol approach is certainly not yet a demonstrated success, (we will await the results of Dr Claire Chilvers' research with great interest). But it never claimed to be a Centre that could cure cancer anyway. And surely, no cancer specialists, orthodox or complementary, really believe that an extended prognosis is the only criterion in judging any treatment's success. Hopefully, all of them these days are equally concerned with enhancing the quality of the patient's life. It is difficult to do that with surgery, drugs and radiation. The chances seem much greater when using the loving medicine that Rosy Thomson describes. But don't let us get dragged into the old orthodox versus complementary debate. There really is no issue. The Bristol specialists never set themselves up in competition with orthodoxy. On the contrary, they do not suggest that conventional treatments should be abandoned. And for their part, many oncologists have been coming to realise that 'social support' (a jargon term that clinicians hide behind, but that roughly translated means 'love and affection') makes their patients feel better and just possibly do better as well.

*Loving Medicine* is about a programme of personal inter-action that results in total transformation in some patients' lives. It is tempting to believe that in these days when psycho-neuroimmunology is the new buzzword, parts of the pro-gramme may reinforce the patient's immune system — reac-tivate depressed lymphocytes, boost the production of immuno-globulins. Bristol does not need to rely upon these unproven theories. The most important part of the transformation is mental, emotional (dare I say spiritual?), rather than a series of possible immune responses.

For this reason, patients who have benefitted from the Bristol regime represent a superb group for anyone interested in notions like vigour, vitality, empowerment and serenity. Rosy Thomson's book gives us just a hint of a process that should be examined in far greater detail, not only for the benefit of cancer patients and their therapists, but for the well-being of other people who aren't really sick, but nonetheless want to be whole.

**Clive Wood,** M.Sc. D.Phil.
Editor of *Holistic Medicine*
(Journal of The British Holistic Medical Association.)

# Introduction

The aims of this book are threefold: –

1. To illustrate the principles of Holistic Medicine, and in so doing to emphasise the need for love, faith, kindness, patience and understanding in the practice of medicine.

2. To begin the process of examination and evaluation of the work of the Bristol Cancer Help Centre. This will be done anecdotally, in the form of a series of case studies. Whilst the results of more rigorous scientific trials are awaited there is an urgent need for a book which will answer both doctors' and patients' questions about the scope of therapy offered and the sorts of results being achieved.

3. To emphasise the similarity of our plight as human beings, whatever roles we play and whatever form our suffering may take, in order to encourage others to follow the example of these cancer patients in actively working towards finding a state of peace, aliveness and happiness.

The book is written for doctors, nurses, patients and indeed anyone who may find themselves trapped within a role, (or roles) which prevent them from expressing themselves fully as individuals. The compromises and limitations of our roles may be so enormous that they almost completely eclipse our true natures. As we lose the power to express ourselves and are unrecognised, we atrophy and the quality of our life, energy, health and work reflects this starvation process. In this state of diminished aliveness we are very prone to disease and unhappiness. This may manifest in some as a kind of creeping melancholia which can drive a person further into self-destructive behaviour, or in others as minor aches and pains, but for yet others the life crushing process is so severe that it results in life threatening disease. However great or small the signs, if we take heed of them, we may be able to give ourselves the jolt we need to wake up and take a good look at ourselves in order to see what games we are playing and to whose rules. The greater the jolt, the more fuel there is for change. When we discover that a particular role is having a deadening effect on us we have two choices — we can either diminish our commitment to that role in order to express more of ourselves outside of it or, better still, confront the fear which is keeping us trapped and limited. As we consciously embrace this fear we find ourselves freer and freer to express ourselves within any situation, especially in our relating to others, be they friends, lovers or patients.

As I went through my medical training, to my great dismay, I found this stunting process to be occuring. I was taught to be responsible, serious and self-important. I was taught to be authoritarian, distant and in control. I was taught that I must always have an answer to every question and that I must fight for the preservation of life in all circumstances. I was taught through my intellect and memory, and given formulae and rules to work to in all situations. The more solidly cast I became within this mould, the less real contact I was able to have with the patients. As I walked into the hospital it was as if the individuality and aliveness drained out of me and I slipped into a grey lack-lustre version of myself. I felt as if there was a plate glass window between me and all the other people or as if we were all on a strange wavelength which wasn't quite tuned into reality. I couldn't talk with the patients about their pain and fear and in so doing enable them to grieve for their lost organs or passing lives. I couldn't hold a patient who was trembling with fear. I couldn't respect the wishes of a patient who did not wish to be resuscitated if he died. I couldn't even give new parents ten minutes peace to drink in the joy and wonder of the birth of their child.

The other side of the coin was the patients' predicament. Implicit in their role was lack of power and knowledge, the unacceptability of the expression of anger, fear or grief and the tacit absorption of and compliance with medical 'truth'. So often under the well behaved, model patient exterior I could sense the raging confusion being experienced by patients receiving very grave diagnoses, or being told they had to undergo a serious operation. I could see us all, doctors, patients and nurses, moving round each other in the impenetrable armour and safety of our roles, glad at one level to be spared a headlong collision with the reality of the pain and grief, but at another level saddened and frustrated by our inability to reach out to each other. After all, most of us who have entered the caring professions have done so out of a desire to express our love and concern for others and paradoxically we find ourselves progressively less and less able to do so.

I was beginning to think I might have to leave medicine altogether as I could see no way out of this trap. A few specific incidents had really horrified me summing up the numbness and emptiness of the practice of medicine. One incident particularly illustrates the way that my natural behaviour was not considered acceptable. One weekend I had been on duty covering a leukaemia ward as a medical house-officer. I had received no special advice about what to expect. A young man called Peter came in on the Friday evening with minor abdominal symptoms, but the results of his blood tests revealed that his leukaemia was out of control. By Saturday evening after intensive treatment he appeared to be much better. At this stage I had met his young wife, mother and father, in-laws and brothers and sisters. We were all trying to cheer each other up and be as positive as possible. Tragically however, our best efforts failed and on Sunday Peter had a brain haemorrhage. The staff nurse who was on that day was a very special woman called Ann. Together we stayed in Peter's room along with about ten members of the family until Peter finally died at around 6pm.

The support we all gave each other was wonderful. They, without speaking, helped me cope with my feelings of impotence and inadequacy, and Ann and I tried to help each of them through their disbelief and grief at losing their son, husband and brother. We all cried our tears and made many journeys back and forth between the Visitors' room and Peter's room to reaffirm the reality of what had happened and say our farewells to Peter. Several hours later we all became more peaceful and the family gathered themselves and left. Of course there were other patients on the ward whose needs had to be attended to by that stage. As I made my rounds, the mother of one of the children with leukaemia called me over and thanked me profusely on her own behalf and on behalf of some of the other parents who had been there during the afternoon. She said that I was the first staff member that any of them had ever seen cry on that ward and that they were deeply relieved that one of us was able to share their grief.

When my evening duties were completed I was summoned by the ward sister to discuss my appalling handling of the situation! She had been horrified at the way I had completely "lost control" of both myself and the relatives. It had been shocking that I had "allowed" so many people to witness the death and it was very reprehensible that this had meant that everyone else on the ward had known what was going on. In the morning her sentiments were echoed by my medical colleagues. I was stunned and upset and retreated back behind the plate glass. I was told that once I had done all I could have done medically, I should have explained the situation to the relatives, making it clear that only two relatives could be in his room at any time and then I should have left. The nurse would have informed me when the death had occured and I would have been called to write a death certificate. There would have been no fuss and no bother.

How could I have assumed that sort of control? What right did I have to shut out the majority of the family if that was where they wanted to be? How much use would I have been to them or to the staff-nurse or myself safely tucked away in my room? The word compassion is derived from Latin and means 'to suffer with'. I know that in my opinion, the opinion of Peter's family and those other parents on the ward, I was infinitely more helpful to them stripped of my mask, suffering alongside them, than I ever could have been in my impersonal doctor's role.

It became very hard to keep swimming against the tide, feeling miserable within this straightjacket. It was strange too, to be mocked by my colleagues for the importance I placed on the humanitarian element in medicine, whilst seeing all around me just how unhappy so many doctors, nurses and patients are within their roles. I was seeing more and more patients turning to alternative medicine to get the attention they really wanted, and was at the same time aware that the medical profession has the highest rates of suicide, alcoholism, drug abuse and other mental health problems of any professional group.

I thought very seriously about whether I might be happier working within the alternative medical world and considered training as an acupuncturist, but had a nagging feeling that this was rather like abandoning the sinking ship; the ship that the majority of the population was on too. To go off into a small private medical niche did not really seem to be the answer. However the urge to explore alternative avenues was strong. There had to be a way of getting a better quality of attention to the patients. So whilst still working within the N.H.S. I set up an Alternative Therapy Centre to which patients could come for hour long appointments to see practitioners of many different disciplines. This was exciting and it was good to get feedback from patients who said that they felt as if someone had finally listened to them after all these years. However, I was very aware that as medical adviser to the Centre 'patients' were still pushing me into the role of doctor, looking to me for the answers, strength, energy and power to cure them. This was an enormous responsibility, not to mention absolutely exhausting. I knew that I could not keep it up for long and that I was doing something wrong. I needed guidance.

It was at this stage that I heard of the formation of the British Holistic Medical Association.* My relief was enormous. Here was an organisation which was founded by a group of doctors who recognised the inter-relatedness of mind, body, spirit and environment in the causation, diagnosis, experiencing and treatment of disease. But more than that, they supported the belief that individuals hold within themselves both the greatest insight into their illness and, given adequate support, the greatest power to do something about it.

I was also excited because the Association had both a lay associate membership and a sister association of complementary practitioners, nurses and all other para-medical groups (The British Association of Holistic Health). The organisation in its broader form therefore comprised a collection of individuals with a common interest in health, who were prepared to dis-regard their roles and meet on an equal footing to find out how they could really best help each other and those whom they served in their work.

I was delighted — at last I was going to meet some kindred spirits within medicine. I went to the Association's 2nd annual conference at Oxford full of anticipation and was not disap-pointed. The two topics under discussion were birth and cancer.

*British Holistic Medical Association, 179 Gloucester Place, London, W.1

As I had rather fancied myself as Britain's answer to Michel Odent I was extremely keen to hear about the Active Birth Movement and rather hoped I might meet a progressive obstetrician who would take me under her wing! I was taken by surprise then to find that what really caught my attention was the work of the Bristol Cancer Help Centre. I went along to a workshop given by one of the Centre's doctors on imaging with cancer patients. I became fascinated. Here was an existing unit putting holistic medical principles into practice. There were doctors, nurses, patients, counsellors, dieticians, healers and art therapists all working side by side. I felt that studying and working at the Centre could really give me insight into how to adjust my attitudes and practice so that I would be a far more effective practitioner and a much healthier individual.

If I have given the impression so far that my main frustrated need was to be involved in high emotional drama that is misleading. I wanted to be able to be both appropriate and loving with my patients. I also wanted to be able to step outside the limitations of the scientific medical model with its hope destroying prognostications, and explore the creative options and transformational possibilities within illness and within the doctor-patient relationship; to find the chinks of light in the darkest moments and by focusing on these rather than gloom, fear and despondency help restore hope, faith, joy and health. But most of all I wanted to offer a haven within my care, enabling people to feel safe enough to relax, grow strong again and find the courage to make the changes necessary for health to return. By being true to my own needs then, I hoped to escape the deadening effect of falling into the conventional doctor's role and feel alive and satisfied. How many of us limp along through life knowing full well that we are working and living at a tenth of our potential, feeling more dead than alive, always waiting for our moment to come (or worse still having given up the hope of it ever coming)? Mercifully though, unlike these cancer patients, most of us are presented with opportunities to wake up without having our lives threatened.

I arranged to visit the Centre and met the co-founder Pat Pilkington, an extraordinarily warm and dynamic woman, who I immediately sensed was at the organisational and spiritual core of the Centre, along with her delightful husband Canon Christopher Pilkington. They welcomed me with open arms and arranged for me to attend the Centre on a weekly basis to observe and participate in their work.

It is fascinating how once off familiar territory we cling to what we know. In my early sessions at the Centre I found myself falling back into my old role of being authoritarian and 'in the know'. I have also seen many patients at Bristol initially clinging to their patient role, being most comfortable at the point in the day when they were given their prescription for vitamins, despite having come to the Centre for an altogether different approach! However over the weeks I began to loosen up, learning from the readiness of others to expose themselves completely whilst in the painful processes of self-examination, re-evaluation of lifestyle, work and relationships; and in the expression of long held-in grief, anger, pain, loneliness, shame and fear of inadequacy. I witnessed the fear and defensiveness as the layers of 'role armour' came off, but also the heady exhilaration and aliveness experienced on finally coming up for air out of the suffocating self-made prison. For some patients reaching this turning point created massive upheavals in their external life, and for others the major change was in their inner lives. Many, having exploded the myths of their own personal nightmares, were discovering an entirely new sense of peace and well-being and often simultaneously experienced partial or complete remission of their symptoms. This process is quite often referred to as 'transformation' for obvious reasons.

The doctors and counsellors at the Centre guided and supported me throughout the year that I visited regularly and encouraged me to believe in myself. I also received great affirmation from the patients who really appreciated my open way of working with them. I became able to accept and value myself and lose my fear of expressing myself. In other words, the Centre helped do for me exactly what it was doing for its patients.

I was struck by the fact that although extraordinary things were happening to people at the Centre, very little had been written about the kinds of experiences people were having there. This, I feel, is reflective of the attitudes of those who work at the Centre; that is non-competitive and without the need to prove anything to anyone. This lack of information about what can be achieved through the Centre's approach seemed to be an omission to me for many reasons. For a start, everyone complains about only ever hearing bad news. I had seen people and heard stories in the Centre which were almost too good to be true. I wanted to share these stories. Secondly, I wanted those who are suffering everywhere, and specifically cancer patients and their families to know about the approach of the Centre so that they might benefit from it directly or indirectly. But almost the most impelling reason of all for writing the book was my desire to communicate with other doctors and health care workers, to give them food for thought about their own practice and lifestyles.

Of course the Centre is aware of the demand of the medical profession for proof where any claim of cure has been made. For this reason they have invited Dr Claire Chilvers of the Marsden Hospital to set up a scientifically water-tight prospective trial funded by the Imperial Cancer Research Institute. This study will compare the survival time of breast cancer patients attending the Centre with matched patients who are not. It is also hoped that another study will shortly be initiated to try to assess some of the subtler aspects of success, e.g. the quality of life of patients attending the Centre as compared with those who are not. The results of these studies may take years to come out however, and the collecting of truly scientific data will be fraught with enormous difficulties. (This will be discussed in more detail in the final chapter.) In the meantime there seemed to be a place for a series of anecdotal case studies to acquaint practitioners with the sort of results being achieved; to clarify where the Centre stands with regard to conventional therapy and to explain the Centre's position on the possible relationship between its therapy and the remission/cure of cancer. I have included, where possible, both objective case details and the comments of the medical practitioners outside the Centre who are involved with each case.

Whilst working at the Centre, I have of course learnt practical techniques and much factual information about alternative cancer treatments. But most important of all I have been given the necessary support and encouragement to begin to be comfortable and confident enough to express my loving nature in my work, rather than working from a base of fear and defendedness. This is the message you will hear over and over again in the stories of the patients: that while the individual therapies have given them useful props at certain times and may have genuinely helped achieve stabilisation of their physical condition, the most important factor in the achieving of health has been the finding of and expressing of their true natures, which has been made possible by the support, love and encouragement provided by the Centre. The beauty of this for me is that having received this support and encouragement myself I now feel ready to go back into the N.H.S. under option two. In other words I am sincerely hoping that I will not have to leave medicine to be myself. I can keep trying to dissolve the boundaries of my roles and express my true nature wherever I am, as I did naturally before at the most special occasion of Peter's death. For this encouragement, increased confidence and greater aliveness, I am eternally indebted to all the wonderful brave people I have met at the Centre.

From the inability to leave well alone:
From too much zeal for what is new and contempt for what
   is old
From putting knowledge before wisdom, science before art,
   cleverness before common sense;
From treating patients as cases and
From making the cure of disease more grievous than its
   endurance,
Good Lord, deliver us!


*Sir Robert Hutchinson 1871-1960*
   *(Past President, the Royal Society of Physicians)*

# PART 1

## Chapter 1

# An Overview of the Bristol Cancer Help Centre

## The History of the Centre

The Bristol Cancer Help Centre was opened in 1980 in a private house. It was the brainchild of Penny Brohn, Pat and Christopher Pilkington and consultant physician Dr Alec Forbes. Penny had been found to have cancer and, despite the lack of any example to guide her, became utterly convinced that her disease was a disease of all of her and not just her left breast. She was therefore equally convinced that her recovery depended on far more than the amputation of her breast. Her conviction was so strong that initially she refused all but a diagnostic biopsy and set off on an agonising journey to find her healing. This search took her to metabolic clinics in Europe and Mexico, counsellors, monasteries, spiritual healers, and biofeedback experts, as well as back to orthodox medicine for tamoxifen and a lumpectomy.

Eight years on, Penny is still very much alive with three grown up children, an extremely enriched marriage, and an acupuncture practice, as well as continuing to work tirelessly as a director and staff member of the Centre. She has also written two books about her experience of cancer and the work of the Centre[1] and made countless T.V., radio and other public appearances to encourage other cancer patients and their families. She had a local recurrence of her cancer four years ago, but to the amazement of her doctors the tumour has stopped growing and she has no secondaries. Her progress is being closely monitored by the radiotherapy department of the Charing Cross Hospital. The most difficult part of her experience was that she had no example to follow and no contact with others who felt the same way. As if this wasn't bad enough she encountered terrific resistance, criticism and anger from those close to her who thought she was being incredibly selfish and engaging in a kind of protracted suicide. Her overwhelming concern then, on having stabilised her own health, was to set up a centre to support and guide others who wanted to make the same journey.

During Penny's stay in the German clinic of Dr Josef Issels she had been visited by her very close friend Pat Pilkington. They spent a lot of time discussing the possibilities of a centre in Bristol. Pat and her husband, Canon Christopher Pilkington, had already been running a healing group in their parish, which they saw as a very important aspect of their work. The setting up of a healing centre was therefore a relatively natural (if rather ambitious and unexpected) progression for them. They quickly became inspired by Penny's ideas and decided to support her in making her dream a reality. By incredible coincidence, soon after her return from Germany, Pat received a letter from Dr Alec Forbes, a retiring consultant physician from Plymouth. He had heard about their healing work and was looking for a setting to put some of his ideas about the Holistic treatment of cancer into practice. The Centre had been born.

It started off running just one day a week with everyone working voluntarily, but was soon running three days a week to meet the growing demand. The charity of those involved was being stretched to the maximum and so was the available space. By this time the Centre had had to call in other doctors, counsellors, dieticians, cooks and many other voluntary helpers to cope with the work load. The last straw was the T.V. series 'A Gentle Way With Cancer' which brought floods of people to the Centre's doors, often from abroad. There had also been requests for residential facilities as day visits didn't seem long enough for some of the patients to gather and assimilate all the information they needed.

Far from being unique, it appeared that Penny's feelings and words had found terrific resonance in patients everywhere. There was nowhere else to send this overflow of patients and no-one involved had the heart to turn them away, so the decision was made to buy large permanent premises to house the Centre. This involved raising an enormous loan, thereby putting the Centre and its staff under a very great strain, which was only eased after three years and monumental fund raising efforts. The saddest part of this move was that it became inevitable that most patients would have to pay for their visit. (There is a bursary fund for patients who cannot afford the fee.) This is entirely contrary to the principles of most of those involved in the work of the Centre but has become the reality of the situation. The Centre now has a staff of around forty people and an enormous building to maintain. This situation may change again in the future if the Centre receives sufficient outside support. It is first and foremost a charity and not a business.

## The Medical View of the Centre

The existence of the Centre has opened up some very difficult dilemmas for doctors, both with regard to its reflection on their own performance and their concern for their patients. The failure of the medical profession to recognise and provide for the emotional, psychological and spiritual components of illness has driven patients to seek help elsewhere often at the price of rejecting conventional treatment altogether. It is outside the comprehension of many doctors, and certainly outside the terms of the Hippocratic oath, that a sense of control, understanding and peace could be more important than 'life at all costs'. Many patients who attend the Centre say that they would rather face their illness and their death than medical treatment and the patient role. This is a horrifying indictment of the state of medical practice. Doctors who may have already been depressed and frustrated by their inability to cross the humanistic gulf are now having their methods and scientific truths questioned and thus their whole raison d'être challenged. This has created a mixture of reactive aggression and dismissal, and very genuine interest in the work of the Centre. Doctors have found themselves both extremely anxious that patients attending the Centre may be causing themselves to die prematurely while at the same time having to acknowledge that many entirely unexpected recoveries have taken place.

It is therefore necessary then that urgent communication be set up so that the best of both worlds may be achieved and mutual trust and education be established. This, in fact, is the major aim of this book. I hope that by explaining both the Centre's stance with regard to orthodox medicine and its views on the possible relationship between its therapy and the remission/cure of cancer to put the minds of both doctors and patients at rest. By describing the therapy and the way in which it is adjusted to meet the needs of each individual, I hope to allay fears that the therapy is dangerous or that any patient is forced into any course of action which does not feel absolutely right for them. But most important of all I hope to help doctors and other health care workers to understand what it is which causes patients to turn their backs on orthodox medicine in search of other therapies, even if this means putting their lives on the line.

## The Centre's Stance with regard to Orthodox Treatment

No patient attending the Centre is ever encouraged or advised to refuse orthodox treatment. Patients often come to the Centre in a state of turmoil about whether or not to have the orthodox medical treatment offered to them. There are many different reasons for this confusion. It may be the fear of side effects or pain. It may be the fear that if they have an organ removed, especially electively (i.e. the spleen in the treatment of Hodgkin's disease or the ovaries in the treatment of breast cancer) that they will never be whole again. Often patients fear that radio-, chemo-, or steroid therapy will badly damage their immune system, which they know is already faulty or depressed in some way. Other patients may just feel completely out of control of their situation and resent the assumption that they should submit to whatever treatment is suggested. Patients are often told and not asked about the treatment they will receive and very little time is spent explaining the treatment or its expected side effects. The difficulty for others is that they have had relatives with cancer and have become painfully aware of the inability of the medical profession to know where to stop. They have seen and helped relatives face gruesome treatment regimes which have often failed to produce the hoped for results, and have weakened or created further problems in the patient, leaving them completely incapacitated and utterly dependent on intensive medical care.

The aim of the Centre's doctors is to counsel the patients about their medical anxieties; to hear out their grievances and try to explain exactly what is being offered by the medical profession and why. Attempts are made to understand and empathise with the patient's point of view, the aim being to support the patient in an unbiased way in the making of an informed decision. Offended patients are also encouraged to appreciate the difficulty of their doctor's role and where necessary to forgive them for their insensitivity. This approach helps patients out of the victim/blaming role and can often re-open communication with their doctors, which is of course vital. Whatever the patients' decision, the Centre will continue to support them, recognising their right to have final control over their own life and body. Where orthodox treatment is chosen, (by far the most common decision), ways are sought to minimise the side effects and help patients undergo this treatment as positively as possible. Where treatment is refused, support is given to face the potential consequences and to reconcile family and friends to this decision. The benefit of this approach is that patients have the great psychological boost, whichever way they have chosen, of feeling completely in control and that they are doing the right thing for them. Because of the non-judgemental nature of the support, they have the option at any time to change their minds without any loss of face.

This line is not often taken within orthodox medicine because of the assumption that patients cannot know or fully understand all the factors involved in the making of an informed decision. This is a fallacy. It is remarkable how quickly people become informed when their life or health is at stake. The issue is that patients are conditioned not to want or expect to have this sort of control or self-determination. If this were not the case, doctors would be able to let go of some of the responsibility of their role, but would of course also lose some of their power.

The lack of time allocated for medical counselling within the orthodox system reflects how little the patients' feelings and emotional state are taken into consideration. Patients will often agree to treatment once they understand it and do not feel backed into a corner. In all the medical counselling I have ever done I have heard the same complaint again and again, that no-one ever explained anything and that no-one listened: no-one attempted to 'get inside their skin' and feel what it was like to be them. I know this is not entirely true because doctors often spend time explaining things to patients, but they fail to allow for the fact that initially patients are almost completely deafened by their fear and that the information takes time to sink in and become assimilated. The cancer may have been present for months, but as soon as it is diagnosed decisions about treatment are often made the same day. Therefore the patient sometimes has to cope with both the diagnosis and major surgery within hours of each other. No wonder patients are left in a state of shock and grief. It is for many as if they have been violated and physically assaulted, because they never really consciously understood and consented to the procedure.

Far from aggravating the grievances between patients and their doctors or the rift between orthodox and complementary medicine, the Centre's doctors do their best to improve relations. They support the patient's own doctor by going over medical information and often support patients in their return to orthodox treatment. They also teach patients techniques to make their treatment more bearable. Part of the principle of holistic medicine is to be open to all approaches, and this includes orthodox medicine.

## The Possible Connection between the Centre's Therapy and the Remission/Cure of Cancer

Patients attending the Centre are told that there is no promise of cure associated with its therapy. The function of the Centre is to help patients achieve their best possible state of health. Cancer patients are often told that not only is there nothing the medical profession can do to help them, but also that there is nothing that they can do to help themselves. This is a very damning statement and far from the Centre's experience. Most people find when they take a good look at themselves, that they are compromised at almost every level. There are many ways that they can make inner and outer changes which release energy and undiscovered potential. Although the exact physical mechanism involved is not understood, it is often observed that the increased sense of aliveness that accompanies these exciting changes is associated with a profound improvement in physical health. The Centre also aims to restore the patients' belief in their own power and to support them in their search to find their true self or healing. The result is that almost everyone who embarks whole-heartedly on this path benefits in some way. Most patients experience an improvement in their physical symptoms and a few patients' cancer disappear altogether. Almost all patients report an improvement in their mental state and ability to cope and when death has become inevitable, where possible, patients and those close to them are helped to approach it consciously, with peace, lightness and dignity. The relatives of those who have died are encouraged to maintain their contact with the Centre until they feel quite ready to let go.

## The Principles underlying the Centre's Therapy

1. That the functioning of body, mind, emotions and spirit are completely inter-related and therefore improvement in the state of health at any of these levels will improve the state of health of the whole person, and,

2. That anything is possible (or certainly where there is a will there is a way).

Of course the second of these statements is completely unjustifiable — you either do or do not believe in miracles. The first, however, is becoming easier to justify. For example, there are now volumes of data on the connection between what we eat, the diseases we become prone to and how dietary manipulation can vastly improve many physical conditions. There is also much subjective evidence of the way in which different foods affect one's state of mind and actual evidence that certain food additives (e.g. tartrazine, the orange colouring in food and drinks), cause abnormal behaviour in children. There is also evidence that exercise changes our neuro-endocrine balance and that the prescription of jogging has been found to be as effective in the treatment of depression as anti-depressant medication. The newly emerging field of psycho-neuro-immunology is rapidly demonstrating the connection between mood/ psychological state and the state of our immune or defence systems. These scientists have also demonstrated the power of thought in the changing of so called unchangeable bodily functions.[2]

During the six years that the Centre has been running there has been a large and constantly changing input of ideas from the patients and staff. The outcome of this is that practically all known methods of improvement of health are taught to the patients. Some of these are aimed at improving the general condition while others are specifically directed at the treatment of the cancer. As well as undertaking various therapies, patients also have the opportunity to discuss and share their ingenious ideas about how to cope creatively with the extremely difficult practical problems their illnesses create.

For ease of classification I will divide the therapies into those aimed primarily at the levels of body, mind and spirit, on the understanding that therapy at any level will affect all the others. In some cases it is very difficult to allocate a therapy in this way because it obviously affects more than one level e.g. relaxation and meditation.

Therapy offered at the Centre can therefore be divided into:-

**Physical** ... Diet, Exercise, Relaxation, Breathing, Vitamin and Mineral Supplementation, Bach Flower Remedies, and occasionally Herbal and Homoeopathic Remedies.

**Emotional/Mental** ... Counselling, Visualisation or Imaging techniques, Directed Imagination, Art Therapy, Group discussion for both patients and relatives or friends, Bio-feedback (as an aid to relaxation).

**Spiritual** ... Meditation, Healing, encouragement of connection with nature and other sources of uplift and joy, e.g. music, loving relationships or formal religious communion where appropriate.

Not everyone continues with all the forms of therapy, and indeed patients are encouraged to use their own discrimination and intuition in choosing a treatment schedule for themselves to undertake at home (although care is taken to ensure that this does not mean avoiding the difficult parts!). Likewise the therapy offered by the Centre is under constant review as this is such a rapidly developing field. As the Centre itself matures new wisdom is emerging all the time and so changes are often made in the programme. There are no set rules at all about what is best and every patient's needs are assessed individually.

## The Physical Therapies
### Diet

Some of the alternative cancer therapy centres around the world
have concentrated on the use of diet as the sole therapy, with
some notable success.[3] It is difficult, however, to ascertain
whether these successes are due to the diets per se or to the
whole hearted commitment to recovery. The diet recommended
by the Centre is not seen as a treatment for cancer, but more as
a sensible synthesis of what is known to constitute a healthy diet
and what is known to tax the body least in terms of both
digestion and homeostasis, whilst omitting anything which
there is good evidence to suspect might be carcinogenic.

This means that patients are encouraged to eat a wholefood
vegetarian diet incorporating plenty of raw food in the first
three months. This automatically raises the fibre content of the
diet. They are discouraged from eating meat, dairy products
(other than yoghurt), salt, sugar, excess fat, and any food
additives or preservatives. All food (where possible) should be
organically produced (i.e. not contaminated with fertilisers,
sprays or drugs). Calories are made up between meals with nuts
and dried fruit. Where necessary protein is supplemented with
high protein drinks and fish, eggs or chicken. Most patients
relax their diet to incorporate these foods after the initial three
month spring cleaning diet. Special care is taken to modify the
diet for those who are rapidly losing weight or who have dietary
difficulties due to extensive gut surgery. Surprisingly, many
people find raw food to be easier to digest than cooked food and
that after a readjustment period it has eased their gastro-
intestinal problems rather than worsening them. A book containing the Centre's newer dietary guidelines and many recipes
has been compiled by Saddhya Rippon, who was the kitchen
administrator until 1988.[4]

Almost everyone who tries this regime, whether a patient or
not, feels an improvement in health. This is experienced as an
increase in energy, stamina, and a feeling of lightness. Apart
from the improvement in morale this boost of energy gives,
many patients also feel that the diet has vastly improved their
body's tolerance of radio and chemotherapy. Those who have
undergone treatment before and after the diet have said that
their side effects have been far fewer and that they are certain

that this is not just due to their psychological improvement. The other very important function of the diet is that initially it is the most tangible part of the therapy, enabling patients to feel that they have begun to take control of their situation. Perhaps most significant of all is that the bodily and mental changes which accompany this change of diet show people that aspects of themselves which they considered to be fixed are not. Therefore the power to change all other aspects of their functioning may be within their grasp. One problem with the diet is that many cancer patients are severe self-stressors with very low self-esteem and often the puritanical and pernickety elements of the diet can feed their neurotic and self-deprivatory tendencies. Sometimes the diet becomes unsuitable for these reasons and it may even be advisable to prescribe a diet which includes lots of treats!

## Exercise

The benefits of physical exercise are obvious and well publicised. Patients may need guidance as to the form of exercise which is the most appropriate for them. It is usually advisable to guide patients away from the more competitive, strenuous and muscle-binding types of sport into more gentle and creative forms of exercise. Yoga, if practised properly, exercises all the muscles, joints and glands in a very balanced way and is therefore encouraged. It also lays excellent foundations for the learning of relaxation and meditation. Swimming is often good for the physically debilitated as the water supports the body while allowing a free range of movements. Tai Chi is also an excellent form of gentle exercise which, like yoga, brings the student into a meditative state. Many of the patients enjoy creative movement sessions at the Centre where they are encouraged to drop their inhibitions and express themselves through movement. This can easily (and less embarrassingly) be continued in the privacy of one's own home!

## Relaxation

Relaxation involves the releasing of tension from the physical body. It is mainly taught by getting the patient to focus sequentially on parts of the body from head to foot, or vice versa, consciously letting go of any tension he or she may find there. This can be aided by a guide or partner who talks the person through the relaxation, simultaneously laying their hand gently and soothingly on the part on which attention is being focused. Many people find a state of deep relaxation easiest to achieve after exercise. This and many other relaxation techniques have been found to have profound physiological and psychological benefits.

Psychologically, people find themselves better able to cope with their pressures and physical pain, and also describe a sense of great well-being. Physiologically, a mass of observations have been made, amongst the most significant of which are reductions in blood pressure and circulating catecholamines (chemicals secreted in response to stress).[5] This in turn causes a reduction in steroid secretion (specifically cortisone), with the removal of its inhibitory effects on the immune system. The stress reaction in the body which results in the release of these chemicals is normally protective, but it is thought that the prolonged stress associated with 20th century living, with all its insecurities, never allows the body's chemistry to return to a state of equilibrium, thereby creating an unhealthy internal environment in which the immune system is chronically depressed. Relaxation techniques, if practised regularly, provide an antidote to this (although not as good an antidote as changing the external environment by identifying and removing causes of stress).

### Breathing

The state of a person's breathing gives an extremely sensitive reflection of their emotional and psychological state. By teaching patients to observe their breathing, they can have an instant guide as to how they are reacting in a given situation. When the breath is controlled in certain ways, eg. slowed and lengthened, the body assumes the physiological state which would naturally accompany that sort of breathing. This in turn brings with it the concomitant state of mind. In other words if one starts to breath in a slow and controlled fashion the heart rate slows, the blood pressure drops, the body relaxes and fairly quickly one feels more relaxed mentally. Similarly a panting breath can be very cleansing and invigorating. The detailed yogic science of breath control is called pranayama.[6] However, great benefit can be gained by learning a few simple techniques alone. Cancer cells are also known to die in the presence of high concentrations of oxygen. It has therefore been hypothesized that deep breathing is not only good for the body and mind but also bad for the cancer.

## Vitamin and Mineral Supplementation

Nutritional research points increasingly to the bizarre paradox that our indulgent Western diets both overfeed and under-nourish us. We take in too much sugar, protein and fat. The levels of sugar, salt and fat in the blood have to be maintained within narrow limits. Therefore when we take in large amounts of these substances the body has to work very hard to achieve equilibrium. This occurs at a price; many vitamins and minerals being needed for the building of the enzymes required in the stabilising process. Much of the 'fresh' food we eat is artificially forced by modern farming techniques for commercial reasons, resulting in food with a poor nutrient value. Much of our food is processed, overcooked, microwaved or frozen with further reduction of vitamin and mineral levels. Thus people eating the average British/European diet are likely to be deficient in many of the vital vitamins and minerals. The Centre's rationale in prescribing vitamins and minerals is to alleviate this chronic deficiency state.

There are theories that cancer cure can be produced by vitamin therapy alone.[7] In some of the alternative cancer therapy centres around the world patients are given mega doses of vitamins in the belief that this will destroy tumours. This is not the practice of the Bristol Cancer Help Centre. There is, however, growing scientific evidence that the anti-oxidant vitamins, A, C and E in reasonable doses have a protective effect by mopping up chemically active free radicals which cause damage to cell membranes.[8] This oxidation process is known to be involved in tumour development and the more progressive orthodox units (e.g. Professor Calman's department in the West of Scotland) are beginning to include these vitamins in their treatment regimes. Vitamin A is given as B-carotene, its non-toxic precursor. Any excess to body requirements is stored in this form and is therefore not harmful to the body. Vitamin B is given for its beneficial effects on the general health and in particular the integrity of the nervous system. It is usually prescribed in the form of Vitamin B complex as there is now evidence that the individual B vitamins are better absorbed in combination with each other and their naturally occuring co-factors.

Mineral supplementation consists of selenium, zinc and occasionally magnesium and calcium. Selenium has been found to be deficient in the soils (and hence the food) of certain areas where cancer incidence is particularly high.[9] Selenium is a constituent of anti-oxidant enzymes and it has been hypothesized that its deficiency limits their production and therefore leaves cell membranes vulnerable. Britain's soil levels of selenium are generally low, hence its inclusion in the Bristol regime. Selenium overload is also known to be unhealthy however, therefore it is given in very small doses. Zinc is given because it is a constituent of enzymes involved in the healing and regeneration of tissues, especially skin and epithelia (lining membranes) which are often involved in cancer. Magnesium and calcium are not thought to have specific anti-cancer effects but are occasionally given when individuals are thought to be in a depleted state.

## Other Medicines used at the Centre

Oil of evening primrose is often given to patients. This is high in gamma-linoleic acid, an important pre-cursor of prostaglandins (which are absolutely basic body chemicals), whose synthesis is blocked by elements in tea, coffee and super-heated fats. It is therefore thought that our normal diet hampers prostaglandin synthesis and that this is another reason for its drain on our overall health. So oil of evening primrose is also given to overcome chronic deficiency states until a healthy diet is well established. A herbal medicine has been concocted for use by the Centre's patients which is both a 'tonic' and 'cleanser'. It is thought to have this effect because of its stimulant effect on the organs of excretion, i.e. liver and kidneys. Many of the Centre's staff are keen on the use of Dr Bach's flower remedies. These, like homoeopathic remedies, are prescribed for each individual according to their personality type, rather than their symptoms. Untrue to this general description but particularly popular around the Centre is the 'rescue' remedy, which can be used to help revive sufferers of emotional or physical collapse.

## Medicines not used at the Centre

Iscador, laetrile (amygdalin), benzaldehyde and coffee enemas no longer form part of the Centre's therapy. It has been felt overall, that in the light of the controversy surrounding their use, the unpleasantness of the treatments and the scanty evidence for their claimed therapeutic benefit, their routine prescription cannot be justified. However, some patients, having weighed up the evidence for themselves, decide to initiate treatment with one or other of these medicines.

Of these the most commonly used by the patients is Iscador. It is an extract of mistletoe and is an anthroposophical medicine. This school chooses their medicines on the basis of the similarity of the plant to the condition they are treating. Therefore it is mistletoe's unruly parasitic tumour like growth and the fact that it fruits when all around is dying that has attracted the anthroposophists' attention. Many patients who use it feel strongly about its benefits. Unfortunately though, to be effective it has to be injected. Its use has now begun to be investigated scientifically with encouraging results. [10]

## The Emotional/Mental Therapies

### Counselling

Counselling is the cornerstone of the Centre's therapy. For many cancer patients their psychological pain or discomfort is worse than their physical pain. Not only do they have to face their own fear of death, disease and treatment, but also an intense feeling of isolation created by the difficulty other people have coping with their situation. Patients often find themselves being kept at emotional arm's length by health care professionals who retreat into the safety of their cold clinical roles. Loved ones quite often unconsciously push patients away too. It is as if the seriousness of the diagnosis makes relatives and friends react as if the patient had died already. The possibility of death means that the dying patient can no longer form a stable pillar of the reality of those close to them. This and other defense mechanisms create a numb barrier between people at the time when they most need love and support. One of the primary functions of the counsellors is to bring people out of this state of solitary confinement and put them back in touch with their feelings and loved ones. This can involve the counsellor in walking hand in hand with that person into 'the valley of the shadow of death' or 'the dark night of the soul' to help them meet their fears. At a simpler level though, it can be a great relief for the patient to just 'be' with someone who is not afraid of them.

The counsellor's role can go a lot further than this however, and great creative use can be made of this very uncomfortable emotional state. The extremely intense emotions which accompany life threatening disease throw a person into a liminal or threshold state in which perceptions and priorities become very different. When there may be nothing left to lose people become much braver and more able to make changes. Petty grievances and destructive patterns can be seen for what they are and there is great motivation to do something about them. Usually, in orthodox settings, this state is not used to benefit patients at all — in fact quite the reverse. Mostly when we experience fear or emotional pain we rush for the sedatives. However, to turn this situation on its head and use this clarity of vision can be of great value to the patient. Breakthroughs may come from the examination and healing of relationships, from the expressing of supressed grief or anger, or the breaking down of the 'coping' facade. With this catharsis can come a great release of psychic energy, as it takes a great deal of energy to keep this difficult material in the subconscious or to maintain the 'shop-front'. The counsellor provides the safe environment and loving support needed for this release to occur.

Another function of the counsellor is to help the person find their 'true self'. At the mundane level this can mean helping them to get in touch with what they really want to do with their time, as opposed to continually doing what they think they should do. This may involve quite unexpected discoveries about careers, hobbies, home and relationships. At a broader level it may mean opening a person to dimensions of themselves that they never knew existed and for the first time opening up the possibility of an inner life. Everybody has an inner life, but our conditioning does not validate it. We can learn ways in which to allow our inner life to nourish us as much if not more than our outer lives.

Most of the Centre's counsellors are strongly influenced by the transpersonal movement in psychology.[11] This psychological perspective combines many of the strands of 20th century psychology (but especially the ideas of Jung, Maslow, Assagioli and Frankl) with aspects of eastern religion, philosophy and psychology. This combined approach allows not only for the psychological self with its connection to the sub- and collective consciousnesses, but also for the higher self with access to universal or divine wisdom and the many gradations of consciousness in between. The acknowledgement and experience of these other levels can be profoundly healing, because they serve to demonstrate the relative reality of our normal psychological level of existence. This can serve to lighten our approach to our individual 'melodrama'. In so doing it can actually break down our intense seriousness and allow humour and levity to return. The entering of the higher self or 'wise observer' part of ourselves or gaining of the transpersonal perspective has been likened to going up a high tower if we want to get a different perspective on the traffic jams below. When we are on the ground in the middle of them they seem like a completely engulfing reality. From the loftier perspective we can see them in the context of the whole, see our way around or out of them and so they lose their power over us.

With the idea that each of us can get in touch with this wise detached observer part of ourselves, goes the assumption that all of us are the real experts on ourselves. There is no special or mysterious knowledge to be attained; it is more a question of getting in touch with what one knows already. Therefore the counsellor's role is to act as a mirror or guide to help facilitate the unearthing of this knowledge. The other assumption in this approach is the universality of the need for love. It is the denial of this need which is the most potent factor in the creation of disease. Thus the cousellor tries to help the individual open herself to the love of their fellow human beings, of herself and of the divine — 'the life force', God or pure love itself depending on one's belief system.

The hardest for almost all of us is to learn to love ourselves. This is often mistaken for selfishness or egotistical behaviour based on massive insecurity. Most of us in this culture actually feel there is something rather obscene or even sinful about loving ourselves. While we are ruthlessly critical of our bodies, looks, achievements, states or moods, we are unable to praise, encourage, nourish or admire ourselves in any way. If we expect anything or anyone else to thrive we do not treat it in this way! Great benefit follows the removing of this barrage of negative messages which can be achieved through the examination and restructuring of self-image. This process can be helped by the reciting of positive affirmations out loud to oneself[12] or by the meditational practice of metta bharvana in which the focus of meditation is the emotion of friendliness or love which can be directed in the meditation towards self as well as others, and indeed all life.[13]

It is also extremely unfashionable these days to have any sort of relationship with the divine — mainly because of the identification of this sort of relationship with religion. It is most of our experience that religion has done far more to separate people than unite them. None the less, living in communion with the life force or God as opposed to seeing oneself as separate, is profoundly nourishing. For those without devotional inclinations the source of this inspiration or connectedness can come through nature, music, human relationships or the joy of creating. We all know the feeling of having our spirit lifted, but rarely seek out the experience.

Usually when we start to love ourselves genuinely, the relating to and caring for other people and our environment becomes much easier. We are less threatened by others, need less from them and can see more clearly the consequences of our actions. In other words, when we are better at loving ourselves we have much more genuine generosity for others. This is because our interactions cease to be so dominated by getting our needs met by them. Once we begin to start being kinder to ourselves and acknowledge our own vulnerability and fragility, it is not a very big jump to realise that the rest of humanity is in exactly the same boat. These changes seem to go hand in hand in this overall softening process and the logical progression is that we become far more compassionate to others.

In these ways then, skilfull counselling can help both remove the dead wood from our lives and help us dramatically enrich and enliven ourselves (mainly by making us brave enough to ask for what we want!). Illness can become an extremely powerful learning experience, and indeed many of the cancer patients who have been through this process have ended up being glad they had cancer. This is because they feel happier and more fulfilled than they ever have done in their lives before. It has certainly been observed at the Centre that the most dramatic recoveries which occur follow big psychological and spiritual shifts.

A few words of warning however. As with other aspects of

therapy, people can use counselling to perpetuate their negative self-view. The positive end of the spectrum is the use of counselling to imbue the illness with meaning. The more negative end is to use it to search for cause and allocation of blame. People extrapolate that, because waking up from a compromised state can vastly improve symptoms, then being the way they are has created their cancer and therefore they, or those close to them, are at fault. The suggestion that we have created our own cancer in this way is a hideous negative self-affirmation and in my opinion completely wrong. It serves to increase guilt and self-loathing. I do not believe cancer to be a creation of the psychological self and I think it is very wrong for therapists to imply this. All people suffer from the same kinds of stresses as cancer patients and not all of us end up with cancer. If indeed we do create our cancer it is at the same level that we create car crashes or thalidamide babies. There is a school of thought amongst those who believe in reincarnation that we create all our experience, however awful, at the karmic or soul level. This may be a useful concept to some people, but as most peoples' focus is on their psychological reality it is difficult for people not to process this in psychological and emotional terms. I have even heard of therapists who have not made this distinction themselves and who have severely stressed patients by insisting that they know the cause of their cancer, in so doing feeding yet another insecurity: that there is some secret or special knowledge of which they are not in possesion.

My personal interpretation of holistic principles is that patients should take responsibility for their health and not their illnesses, using their illnesses purely as a sign that that their life may well be out of balance in some way.

### Visualisation or Imaging

This is a technique which was pioneered by the Simontons in America in their work with leukaemia patients.[14] The underlying principle is to use the power of the mind to help to get rid of the disease. They used an extremely literal approach initially, getting patients to imagine their cancerous cells being destroyed by their immune cells. However, people found this a very difficult image to form and so the Simontons' got them to image the cancer as a cauliflower being gobbled up by pirhana fish (with far better results). This technique was expanded by other cancer patients who began to use all sorts of other images and symbols, but still on the goody/baddy theme. In other words, the patient was encouraged to imagine their cancer in any form that came to them, then to imagine an effective destructive agent systematically removing the cancer from their body. Emphasis was placed on the necessity to completely destroy the cancer every time the imaging was undertaken. Many patients find this kind of technique extremely useful. An interesting side product of this type of imaging are the clues it gives therapists about what may be fundamentally blocking a person as the images used and the feelings experienced by the patient during the imaging process speak volumes about the individual's experience of life. It also can give insight as to the real extent of their motivation and will to live. Exploration of very half-hearted imaging has quite often led to significant counselling breakthroughs. This may also shed light on the possible secondary gains of the illness which are stopping a person from getting well.

At the Centre a less destructive and more gentle type of imaging is preferred. This is sometimes termed transformative imaging. As stated above a large part of the therapeutic approach of the Centre revolves around getting the patients to nourish and love themselves. It therefore follows that they should not really be encouraged to focus hatred on any part of themselves, especially not their wounded part. In this type of imagery, therefore, people are encouraged to think of their own personal healing image. This image should create a feeling of great well-being, peace and wholeness. These images too, can give insight into the condition of the patient. Some patients opt for a combination of both methods, mentally destroying their cancer first and going on to bathe themselves in a healing atmosphere afterwards. Some people have had spectacular remissions of their cancer through the use of these techniques alone.

### Directed Imagination and Art Therapy

Directed imagination involves the same principles as individual imaging, the difference being that a therapist talks a patient or group of patients through a set of images. This can be a good way of helping people who find imaging difficult. The technique can also be used by the therapist in individual sessions. Insight can be gained as clients reveal their reactions to a given set of images. Often in this right brain function activity, information can be gleaned which is hard to elicit from the more guarded left brain (which is active in conventional counselling/psycho-therapy). This theory also applies to art therapy. The idea is to suspend the critical faculty as much as possible and paint what-ever comes. Sometimes a starting point can be to ask patients to draw their cancer. A sensitive and intuitive art therapist can often help a patient get very significant insight from what emerges. However, great benefit may ensue from the self-expressive/play nature of this exercise alone.

**Group Therapy**

Groups of patients meet during their visits to Grove House for discussion rather than encounter. In the early visits this can be one of the most rewarding features of the programme, helping to dispel feelings of isolation. Great comfort is derived from meeting other people with similar problems and feelings. Groups are also run for relatives who are as much in need of support as the patients, in fact sometimes more so. The patient has usually been receiving a lot of attention while the relatives may have been coping completely alone. While the patient is being encouraged to let go of their coping facade, their friends and relatives may be busy building theirs. As well as groups within the Centre, many patients who have greatly benefitted from the therapy have gone away and set up support groups in their own areas. This is a fantastic help and back-up to the Centre's work. Return visits to the Centre are difficult for a lot of patients, who still need regular input, contact and encourage-ment. These groups give the opportunity for patients to pool resources, ideas and contacts but most important of all, to give each other love and support.

## Spiritual Therapy

There is much confusion about the spirit and spiritual matters. Even this title is innacurate as the spirit cannot be ill so much as eclipsed by unharmonious influences. Therefore therapy aimed at the spiritual plane invariably involves the shedding of dead wood in order that we may uncover our basic spiritual nature. We can do this ourselves in the practice of meditation or can be aided into this harmonious state by healers. I find myself wanting to demystify 'spirit', which to some may sound like a contradiction in terms. This urge arises because often the very word elicits feelings of confusion and religious guilt. I believe that it is the part of us which is connected with all life and could be described as our basic energy which manifests physically as our bodies, at subtler levels in our psychic or mental energy field, and at finer levels still as our soul and spirit.

There are some who believe that disease begins at these finer energy levels, eventually manifesting at the coarsest level in the physical body. As stated earlier, I believe that all planes are fundamentally the same energy manifesting at different frequencies. I therefore feel that it is fallacious to perceive mind, body and spirit as different entities and therefore believe that therapy aimed at any level will affect all the others. This applies to both good and bad therapy. For example, therapy which is insensitively applied at the physical level has injurious effects at the psychological and spiritual levels leaving patients feeling emotionally as well as physically bruised.

## Meditation

Meditation is the process of emptying our consciousness of its contents, namely our thoughts, emotions and feelings and focussing our underlying awareness. This practice has been known by many cultures and religions to have profoundly beneficial effects on all aspects of our function, leading to the development of greater and greater insight into our own natures and the nature of life. As with profound physical relaxation where we can lose all sensation of our bodies, a point can be reached in meditation where the input to the brain is so low that all sense of self is lost. During very deep relaxation we lose the sensation of our body because it is so still that the brain has no cues to pinpoint its location, position or state. Similarly in meditation if all thoughts, feelings and emotions cease, how do we know who we are? For most people their mental activity is predominantly undermining, being full of anxiety, feelings of inadequacy and loneliness, self-criticism and negative affirmations. All of these feelings stem from the ego and the perception of oneself as a separated entity. In true meditation there is a genuine break from this barrage of negative influences. A great sense of peace and connectedness ensue, and with much highly disciplined practice a state of pure bliss can be achieved.

As mentioned in my description of counselling, it is as if the experience of this egoless state of consciousness loosens the grip of our obsessive psychological selves — a blessed relief for most people.

In most meditation practices the focussing of the mind is done through the learning of one-pointed concentration. This may involve concentrating on the breath, a sound or mantra, a picture or even a candle[15]. Most people find this process extremely difficult initially. Until trying to quieten the mind, one does not realise just how cluttered and busy it is, and what resistance it will mount! It is as if the ego puts up quite a battle against being dismissed in this way. The Buddhists have clearly defined the 'hindrances' experienced by most people to getting into a meditative state[13] and for anyone who wishes to practice meditation properly it can be of great benefit to do a meditation course with a Buddhist group (which does not need to involve becoming a Buddhist). As with everything, meditation takes time to learn. However the effects become evident quickly if practice is sustained. The major benefits are far greater mental clarity, alacrity, tolerance, peacefulness and detachment. This results in far more rational action and better decision making. There are physiological changes too which accompany meditation, such as the shift to predominantly alpha-brain waves and the favouring of parasympathetic nervous system activity. These changes are known to improve the functioning of the immune system. Its practice cannot be recomended highly enough to the 'well' as well as the 'sick'.

## Spiritual Healing

Healing is the restoration of a state of equilibrium or well-being in an individual through energy transfer. This may be in the form of love, faith, positive thought (either with the recipient present or absent), prayer, or touch. There are many theories as to how healing works, from divine intervention, to psycho-logical manipulation or placebo effect, to channelling of life force or energy from one individual to another, or to the re-aligning or balancing of an individual's own energy. The vital ingredients in whatever system seem to be love (or genuine care), positive intention and faith. The results do seem to vary from the creating (as with meditation) of a sense of integration and well-being to real and measurable physical improvement,

relief of pain, or even disapearance of symptoms altogether.[16]
Many people are alienated by the religious connotations of
healing and paradoxically others feel that it may not be religious
enough! As stated above genuine spiritual uplift can be achieved
in less alienating ways too, from the pure experiencing of love
or joy, sexual union, music, nature and creativity.

## Who Comes to the Centre?

1. Cancer sufferers whose disease was so widespread at
   diagnosis that they were never offered any conventional
   treatment.
2. Cancer patients who have undergone conventional treatment in the past but for whom the disease has now become
   untreatable in conventional terms.
3. Cancer patients with active disease who are currently
   undergoing conventional treatment.
4. Cancer patients who are in remission or who are 'clinically
   clear' after surgery, radiotherapy or chemotherapy.
5. Cancer sufferers who do not want any orthodox treatment
   at all or who wish to be counselled before deciding upon a
   course of action they will take.
6. Friends and relatives of all the above categories.
7. Observers who wish to learn more about the approach.

Patients who present at the Centre do so for a variety of reasons
in vastly differing states of health. Many of those who come do
so as a last resort when orthodox medicine has nothing left to
offer. Most of the patients who are referred to the Centre by
their doctors fall into this category. When this is the case the
challenge is enormous, but so too is the patient's own resolve to
take the situation into their own hands. Often the power of
resurrecting the patient's belief in their own self-healing ability
and mobilising their inner resources is so great that patients
experience a vast improvement in health. This may be sufficient
to keep their condition stable or in some remarkable cases to
cause the complete disappearance of their tumour.

For others who may not be terminally ill and may be in the
process of undergoing medical treatment the therapy has all the
above possibilities as well as being able to help them cope with

the side effects of treatment. Many patients have found that the use of positive imagery whilst undergoing radio or chemotherapy has vastly diminished their adverse effects both physically and mentally. Others have noticed that the diet and nutritional supplementation have made a big difference.

As the Centre has become better known, more and more patients come on first hearing their diagnosis, some in the very early stages of disease. This is obviously the best possible situation, although sometimes the lack of a gloomy prognosis causes people to be far more half-hearted in their approach. Even better still are the requests made to the Centre for advice about cancer prevention. There have even been people who have no cancer at all, who have been so impressed by the effects of the Centre on their friends, that they have asked if they may come too! This is not possible due to limited resources, but it does give an impression of the power of the approach. It is the most pressing current aim of the Centre to set up an educational programme to apply its philosophy and methods to cancer prevention.

The other group of people who come to the Centre are the patients' friends and relatives. One of the most basic principles of holistic medicine is that the patient does not exist in isolation. Just as it is part of the Centre's role to help people look at and understand the effect their environment may be having on them, it is also necessary to take the other half of this loop into consideration. Quite often the state of illness holds terrific secondary gains for the patients, very much at the expense of the people close to them. Even without this element, caring long-term for someone who you love who is in pain or distress is an enormously demoralising task. The sense of impotence, sadness and frustration which develops can actually cause the carers to withdraw or even become quite hostile. Often as death looms closer they may draw back still further, either due to anticipatory grief or because of their own fear of death.

Sharing and discussing these feelings among relatives and friends who come to the Centre can be enormously cathartic and supportive. Just knowing that other people are going through exactly the same insecurities and finding their own weaknesses is an enormous relief. Also helping to spread out the burden by giving patients and their relatives the addresses of support groups countrywide can be a life saver. Of course there is always the potential of the ultimate trauma for the relatives of the death of the patient. As previously mentioned, this is often diminished if death has been approached very consciously and 'unfinished business' has been completed. Many of the patients themselves are strongly convinced that their illness was precipitated by unresolved grief. It is therefore felt that grief counselling of the bereaved will be a vital part of the Centre's cancer prevention programme.

Lastly, the Centre receives an enormous throughput of people who want to learn about the approach and observe work in progress. Visitors may join in with group sessions, try the food, and talk to the patients, relatives and therapists. There are also regular seminars, day courses and workshops for those who want to study and experience the philosophy and techniques. Talking or writing about phenomena is never the same as experiencing it and so the most powerful way to understand the effects of these practices is to try them for oneself. The next best way is to hear the stories and personal testimonials of the patients who have turned their whole experience of life and illness on its head. This is why I have chosen to keep the theory section as short as possible in order to devote the book to attempting to communicate the direct experience of the patients.

## The Book

I have purposely chosen patients for whom the results of adopting this approach to their illness has been profound and transforming. This is because my main aim at this stage is merely to report a most startling phenomenon that I have had the privilege to observe. It is not intended as a presentation of a representative sample of patients attending the Centre. Nor is it supposed to be any sort of research or controlled study. There are conventional trials in progress at the Centre which will provide statistics for those who base their decisions on this sort of data. Of course there are people who come for whom the Centre is no help at all or who find the approach nonsensical or even infuriating. This too is absolutely fine. The Centre is not intended as a universal answer to cancer. In fact the reverse is true, there is no one answer. So it is absolutely predictable by its own philosophy that there will be many people for whom it is an absolute nonsense. By the same token there are individuals for whom the orthodox medical approach is an absolute nonsense. The Centre has its failures but so too does the medical profession. In the meantime I cannot resist the temptation to report these extraordinary cases, as to me they illustrate the immense untapped power of the individual.

The phenomenon reported in this book is relevant to all people who are struggling with feelings of erosion of their power and sense of control. While it would obviously be better to change the environment in which we live, the reality for most of us is that we do have to learn how to cope creatively with situations beyond our control. I hope therefore in the telling of these patients' stories you will learn as much and be as inspired as I have been by the bravery and ingenuity of these incredible people.

Between the long and short case histories of the patients I have included a chapter for the scientists which has been kindly prepared by Dr Michael Wetzler of The Cancer Help Centre. This contains a summary of the historic background and scientific evidence for the role of the mind in both the causation and cure of cancer.

## Chapter 2

# Evelyn Davies
## Medical History
(*Birth Date*: 6 March 1936)

*Submitted by Dr Rees (Evelyn's new GP) and Mr Pollock (Surgeon).*

Evelyn presented to her GP in June 1985 with a lump in the axillary tail of her left breast. She was immediately referred to Mr Pollock, who performed a biopsy while Evelyn was under anaesthetic. Finding the lump to contain adenocarcinoma in its centre, he proceeded to perform a Patey Mastectomy. Axillary lymph nodes biopsied at the time of diagnosis were found to be normal. No other screening tests were performed at the time to look for the presence of secondaries, but subsequently she has had chest, spine and pelvic x-rays, which were all found to be normal, as was a mammograph of her right breast. Because the disease had been found to be so localised she was not offered Radio- or Chemotherapy. She still attends Mr Pollock's clinic for six monthly follow-ups and happily, no evidence of recurrence has been found since her operation.

## Evelyn's Story

Evelyn is a teacher who lives in Powys, Mid Wales. Her husband is a Church in Wales clergyman and they have two grown up daughters. She now believes that her 'illness' has been with her for many years, but it only began to dawn on her how very wrong everything was in 1984. She says, "I was just so stressed — it was as if everything was out of focus. I was irritable and tired and it was a terrible effort to do anything. Rather than look at what was happening, which is what I would do now, I just closed the doors and pitched in, carrying on with my teaching job full time, in fact working harder than ever. I complained that I was over-working all the time, but at the same time I didn't want to think about myself at all. I used to have the radio or television on any moment I was by myself; I couldn't stand to have silence around me. I didn't want to hear my thoughts." It was during that year that she found her breast lump, but that too was just another thing she didn't want to think about. She had had a breast lump about five years earlier which had turned out to be benign, so she decided to ignore this one along with all the other signals she was getting.

This state of affairs went on for about a year until one Wednesday morning she suddenly sat bolt upright in bed and said to herself, "This is absolutely ridiculous — you're going to the doctor right now". She got to the surgery about an hour before it opened and sat waiting for her GP. Both the GP and the surgeon to whom she was referred were very reassuring, telling her that they thought it was benign but that she should have it removed anyway just to be sure. In June 1985 she therefore arranged to take three days out of her hectic schedule to go into a BUPA hospital, fully expecting to be back to life as normal within that short a period. After all, why should this time be any different to the last time? She was shocked rigid then when she came round from the anaesthetic to find herself 'wrapped in barbed wire'. She realised with horror that these strange pains all over her left side meant was that she had lost her breast — she did have cancer after all. Of course the possibility of mastectomy had been mentioned to her and a consent form had been signed, but the chances had seemed so remote that she hadn't even given it a thought. She had in fact been given quite a radical operation, and had had an axillary lymph node clearance as well as having some of the muscular tissue removed. This was extremely worrying for Evelyn because she is left handed and initially found moving her left arm extremely difficult.

After that initial realisation she says that she became quite flat emotionally. She just accepted it. The nursing staff were kind and helpful but there didn't really seem to be anyone around for her to talk to. "There was no-one I could get any sense out of so I just kept quiet". All through the recuperation period, although she received some physiotherapy follow-up to make sure

she would start to use her arm properly again, there was no
mention at all of cancer and certainly no enquiry as to how she
was feeling emotionally. Her reaction to this was to knuckle
down, do everything that she was told and become a 'model
patient'. What this actually meant to her was that she just
switched off completely. It was as if she was running on
automatic pilot. Underneath she now realises that she was
furious at the medical profession for not giving adequate
psychological preparation for this sort of eventuality. She was
not quite fond enough of herself though to face the fact that she
was angry on her own behalf. Her thoughts were, "I've been a
psychiatric social worker, I'm trained to cope with this sort of
thing, but what about all the people who haven't had my sort
of training?"

Without having read a single alternative cancer treatment
book she came to the conclusion herself that she must change
her diet. She had been looking after herself very badly during
that previous year, eating far too much starchy food, so she
immediately put herself onto an extremely healthy diet. The
next thing that happened was that she met someone locally who
was receiving acupuncture. She asked this person to ask the
acupuncturist if there was anything that could be done for her.
The message came back that she couldn't help but that she had
been in college with a woman called Penny Brohn who had
started a centre for cancer self-help in Bristol.

She started to ask around locally to see if anyone had heard
about it and got all sorts of off-putting answers like, "That's the
place where they do funny things with carrots isn't it?" Evelyn
formed a mental image of a centre run by a load of hippies, but
was still not daunted. As she puts it now, "I hadn't had a day
out for ages, so I thought why on earth not give it a try? What
have I got to lose?" She now says that day completely changed
her life. She says, "It was the most uplifting experience I have
ever had, I haven't been the same since. It was absolutely
wonderful."

What it did make her realise, though, was how very much
work she had to do on herself psychologically. She decided her
first task on returning from Bristol was to find 'a helper'. She felt
that her husband, despite being a counsellor and clergyman,
was the wrong person as he was too close. She searched for
weeks through the clergy of Wales to try to find someone and

eventually discovered that Lyn, the vicar of the nextdoor parish was a trained Christian Counsellor! He didn't ever advertise, but had been involved in counselling and the ministry of healing in a quiet way for years. They went right back to Evelyn's birth. As they unravelled her history she was amazed at how much 'unfinished business' she had shelved along the way.

Her mother had died of TB when she was three weeks old, and had never touched Evelyn because of the disease. Shortly after the mother's death Evelyn's eighteen month old sister had also died of TB, and then when she was two her father died of the same disease, so her whole family was wiped out. For the first sixteen months of her life she was passed around her mother's sisters, none of whom really wanted custody of her. Eventually her father's sister reluctantly agreed to take her. This meant that she never felt that she was wanted or part of the family. She felt like an appendage who had been dumped on her Aunt, and that her Aunt was only doing her Christian duty in raising her. They didn't adopt her or change her name and so she was always very obviously the odd one out. She felt as if she didn't belong to anybody. There was one girl cousin, Sheila, with whom she might have been friends but she was nine years older and so she was little consolation to Evelyn.

The result was that she behaved appallingly throughout her childhood, continually testing her foster parents in a desperate attempt to try to get the attention and love she so badly needed. She says that in her teens she became even worse. She did terribly at school and became very unruly and aggressive. A serious contributing factor to this was that no-one had realised that she was dyslexic. So she was punished for not trying, when she was trying as hard as she could. She recalls that she could read and she knew she wasn't thick — it was just the spelling and the writing she couldn't manage. She now specialises in the teaching of dyslexic children as she never wants anyone else to suffer as she did at that time.

One of the things that came up through her counselling was that she had always felt quite consciously that she had to live for three people: herself, her mother and her sister Margaret. This put the most terrible strain on her because it was hard enough living for one. She had had to cope with the conflicting realities that 'she was the lucky one to be alive' while her life was actually complete misery. She was incredibly lonely, she was in trouble at home, in trouble at school and had no friends at all because she just didn't know how to make or sustain relationships. She was very unhappy. The reason she didn't feel she had to live for her father too was because in her fantasy world he had never really died. She made him into a sailor who was away at sea and who might well come back at any moment. Presumably this relates to the ages at which she lost the different members of her family. In developmental terms, by the age of two she would have formed a notion of her father as separate from herself, but would have been too young when she lost her mother and sister to have conceptualised them as individuals. She had seen photographs of Margaret and her mother and had a complex fantasy life revolving around them too. She now thinks that she bonded to her image of her dead family as she never bonded to anyone living.

Once her schooling was over she was so desperate to get out into the world that despite her dyslexia, through 'sheer bloody-mindedness' she got herself to teacher training college and then carried on to do a postgraduate Psychology course and a degree in Special Education. She now believes that if a dyslexic person is determined enough, eventually another part of the brain takes over as the language centre and the problem will eventually fade. While she was at college she got engaged to a very 'unsuit-able' boy. She realises in retrospect that this was really another test or punishment for her foster parents — she had no real intention of marrying him. This was the start of a series of two or three other fairly unproductive relationships. Eventually, when she could stand home no longer, she found a way out through taking up a residential teaching post in what would now be termed a girls' borstal. Evelyn identified strongly with the girls as many of their backgrounds were not dissimilar to her own.

One day her work was abruptly terminated when one of her pupils pushed her down a flight of wooden stairs in a fit of rage. Evelyn was very badly shaken and also had a broken collar bone. She was offered a friend's cottage in Wales in which to convalesce, and she accepted. It was at this point that her life began to sweeten a little. During this convalescence she met and fell in love with her future husband, who was the minister of the parish where she was staying. She never went back to the school and they eventually married. This laid the foundation for a reconciliation with her 'family', and Evelyn ultimately nursed her aunt (the one who had brought her up) at her marital home during the latter's terminal illness. She is now very close to Sheila too. One very liberating moment for Evelyn was to discover that they had actually shared a lot of negative feelings towards her 'parents'. Evelyn had felt guilty about these feelings, seeing herself as most wicked to have these thoughts while identifying Sheila as the paragon of virtue who would never dream of thinking such things.

Evelyn had tried to close the doors on all this unhappiness when she married and started her own family, but she came to realise in her counselling the extent to which her woundedness, anger and guilt had continued to dominate her. She had always refused or been unable to talk about her past. She now realised that the feelings had really festered on all through her adult life, and will even admit the jealousy and resentment she felt towards her own children for having simple happy lives. It took the anger that she felt after her operation to put her fully back in touch with the buried crippling rage that she felt towards her own family for dying, and her foster family and teachers for making her life so miserable. The cancer had finally given her a legitimate outlet for this anger. She says that it was during her very first counselling session with Ludi How at the Centre that she realised that she could open these doors up and let all her pent up feeling out without being damaged still further. Ludi made her feel safe enough to do this.

However, her imaging reflected her sub-conscious resistance to this process. She imaged her cancer cells as being shut into a box with herself sitting on the lid. She saw these cells as red. Instead of the cells dying they seemed to be getting bigger and bigger and it was becoming harder and harder to keep the lid on. What is fascinating is that during this time she became acutely anaemic. It slowly dawned on her that what she was actually doing was sitting on her own strength in some way. So she finally decided that she had to let the lid come off the box. What had been in the box was not her cancer but her red blood cells. With their release came a huge amount of red-blooded anger. With the awakening of this anger she had decided to fight — but for the first time in her life she felt she wanted to fight for herself — not for other people or against other people — just for herself.

This was the most frightening part of the whole process for
her. She did it all by herself at home in bed one night. She
thought that when she took the lid off the box she might be
struck dead immediately. When nothing actually happened to
her physically there and then she was able to laugh at herself in
relief. From that moment onwards the anaemia began to resolve
and she got stronger again. This demonstrated to her not only
the power of visualisation, but also her own power and she felt
enabled to take the process deeper. She was no longer frightened
to face herself and felt for the first time in her life that she could
stop pretending. She realised that from the moment she had
become the 'Parson's wife', she had felt the need to be perfect
in every way. She felt extremely responsible for all around her
and would cripple herself with guilt and anxiety if anything
went wrong, either in the parish or at home. It was all her fault
because she was not perfect enough. Her guilt was in fact so
great that she now realises that when she got her diagnosis she
actually felt, "Ah yes, this is right, this is what I deserve for
being such a bad person — I'm getting my come-uppance now".
Looking at this she realised that this had very old origins. As a
child her foster parents had told her continuously how lucky she
was, and that if she wasn't grateful God would punish her. She
wasn't grateful at all, and while her rebelliousness may have
been her saving grace at the time, there was always the lurking
guilt and knowledge that at some time she would be punished.
So, lying there in her hospital bed, she thought, "Right, this is
it, God is punishing me and now I'm going to die". She took the
diagnosis of cancer as synonymous with death.

Her image changed to one of pure light after letting go of the
box. She sees herself bathed in white light and will direct the
centre of the light to any part of herself which may be
particularly sore on that day.

The other problem she used to have was that initially she was
too frightened to go to sleep at night in case she died in her
sleep. At bedtime now, she images herself beside a cool misty
pool. She has a big bucket in her hand into which she places all
the rubbish of the day. She then tips it into the pool where it
dissolves away. She then watches the ripples gradually disappear, but she says she never sees the end because she is always
asleep by that point. She finds this makes an enormous amount
of difference to how she feels when she wakes. Before she

loathed the mornings, but now she is up and about feeling fresh and happy. This began to happen after she really confronted her own fear of death. After her diagnosis she used to have dreadful nightmares and so was eventually forced to meet her fear head on. She now has completely the opposite feeling describing death as the last great adventure. She feels that it is a gate, not an end or a beginning. She actually looks forward to it now, but knows she has a lot of work to do before she will be allowed that 'privilege'.

The main catalyst for Evelyn, on that momentous day at the Centre which started the whole ball rolling, was simply the feeling she had walking through the door. She said that another dimension which had never been open to her before opened up as she walked into the place. She finds it very hard to put into words, but feels that it was the spirit of love and acceptance. She wasn't the parson's wife, she wasn't the bad girl of the family, she wasn't a teacher and she wasn't a mother — she was just her and it was enough — she felt wanted and safe. The feeling was as if something had just rolled off her back. She says that until it was gone she had never realised it was even there. She describes it as a great lump which was lying across the back of her neck, dragging her down. She thinks it was her guilt — her guilt at actually being alive.

When she went home she was intoxicated with happiness and relief. For the first time in her life she felt that she had as much right as anyone else to be alive. It was permissible to live just for her, and not to have to live for her mother and sister because she wasn't really good enough. She had finally begun to exist in her own right. This feeling of elation and self-confidence lasted, opening the floodgates for the buried hurts to come pouring out. She talked and talked and talked with her husband in a way that had never been possible before. This period was also when she started her counselling with Lyn, which was greatly facilitated by her new aliveness and freedom from old fears. She thinks it is quite funny that she used to get frustrated by her husband's accepting attitude, feeling she had to stir him into action. She now knows he was right all along, and that it has taken her 25 years to get to where he is!

The other big change that came about was that she became fully able to pray. As well as counselling her, Lyn also spent time guiding her in prayer. She had been a Christian all her life, had been a minister's wife and had even taught religious education and Sunday schools. In developing a relationship with herself she had begun to experience an entirely different relationship with the Divine. She says, "Before it was all outside me, I was probably too angry with God to open myself up before, but was much too inhibited to dare even think that". As her faith and ability to enter into true communion has grown, she is more and more amazed at her old self in the role of the parson's wife, desperately concerned about what she was seen to do no matter how switched off she was inside. She says that before all her prayer was one way. She would constantly be talking to God and not listening. She says that now it almost feels as if the top of her head is open and she feels beauty, strength and warmth cascading down her spine when she prays.

Through her illness Evelyn has become integrated into life for the first time. She no longer lives in a lonely anxious prison. Since taking her step into life she has now experienced full relationships with other people. Her relationship with her husband is entirely different. She says, "I've got so much living to catch up on now, there just isn't enough time in every day. There just is no stress in my life any more. I do exactly the same as I did before, but enjoy every minute of it now. It is the most extraordinary feeling because I have never been stress-free in my entire life. I feel like I'm walking on air. I can't imagine how I got through every day before feeling so tense and miserable."

She now feels completely inspired to carry her own experience forward by getting more involved in the Healing Ministry of the Church. She is seriously considering the possibility of formalising her commitment by becoming a deaconess. I asked Evelyn whether this was part of her old pattern, namely, if she has found something good she doesn't deserve to keep it for herself, but has to give it away to others. She says this time it is very different because she feels it can only enrich her own experience. She feels balanced for the first time in her life and that she is now working from a steady base. While all her work will be in the service of others she will be doing it every bit as much for herself. She feels a great urge now to practise healing herself through the laying on of hands, but is holding herself back somewhat at present until she is sure that this is right and that she is strong enough. She also needs to get over the feeling that there is something a bit presumptuous about suddenly deciding she is a healer. Sitting with her I do not think she is being at all presumptuous because her very presence was extremely healing and uplifting for me. She finds now that when she tries to help others who are suffering she uses her imaging to hold an image of Christ between herself and the other person to remind herself all the time that the healing is coming from God and not from her. This she feels protects her from getting sucked in to the other person's hell and from taking on too much personal responsibility.

After I saw Evelyn in July 1986 she was asked by the Bishop of St Asaph to meet Bishop Graham Chadwick who has led her further into meditation and prayer. This has strengthened further 'the base on which she grows'. In September 1986 she found a small cottage in Mid Wales close to a shrine and ancient healing centre. Through an extraordinary set of 'co-incidences' the money became available for Paul and Evelyn to buy this cottage. This will be the first home they have owned. However it is their intention to turn it into a healing centre and retreat house for small groups and individuals. Meanwhile she has set up the Meifod Cancer Support Group which is affiliated to the Bristol Cancer Help Centre and BACUP. The group works on three levels. They operate a crisis telephone counselling line. They provide individual counselling and they run group support sessions. They have received fantastic support locally and funds and offers of help have poured in from as far afield as America! Local GP's are already referring patients to their group and they also see people who do not actually have cancer but who are anxious about getting it. One of the group's projects is to work with the medical profession locally on issues such as how to break the news of terminal illness.

In summary then, the greatest blessing of all for Evelyn is her newfound sense of peace and joy. She does also praise the Centre's diet. She has remained on it for a year and says she's never felt fitter in her life. As well as feeling the effect mentally as a general sharpening of her wits she has really enjoyed the feeling of lightness in her body. This is a real boon for Evelyn as she has been overweight for most of her adult life. She feels that it is important for those who come to Bristol to take on the whole package. She says, "Whether you are 30, 50 or 70 you have to stop everything you are doing and completely start again. It is no good being half-hearted." She feels she has learned more life-skills in the past year than in the rest of her life. She says she is glad that she had the cancerous growth because if she hadn't she would still be a complete mess. She does still come to the Centre regularly because there is a special quality of feeling that she gets there that she cannot really get elsewhere. She feels that her joy and inspiration is topped up.

Despite feeling this, she does think that healing and counselling are transferable into the N.H.S. context. She feels that all patients should be counselled prior to major surgery so that they can really understand what is going to happen and so that they can name their fears and ask any questions. She is sure that this could be done in groups to save counselling time. An advantage of this would be that any fears or constructive ideas would be shared immediately, preventing the sense of isolation before it even began. Any individual embarrassment could be avoided by asking individuals to place their questions into a pot before the group started.

In particular she feels that breast cancer patients should be seen and counselled by women. She knows a woman locally who just couldn't bring herself to go to the doctor for three years with her breast lump because she was too embarrassed to undress in front of him. This is the most extreme example of breakdown of communication. Evelyn feels there are many subtler, traumatic aspects for women undergoing any sort of breast surgery. For many women the feeling of violation they have after an operation such as she had can do lasting damage, often drastically affecting a woman's sexuality and overall confidence. However, the most vital part of any such counselling as far as Evelyn is concerned is that the person be given choice. She had no choice at all as to the timing or type of operation she had and feels badly about this. Her warmest memory of her medical treatment was her session with the sister in the prosthesis (false breast) clinic. She said it was such a relief to be in the hands of a capable friendly woman who wasn't the least bit embarrassed about the job she was doing. Evelyn felt that possibly her role could have been extended to that of counsellor as she was dying to ask her some questions but the woman was just too busy.

Evelyn never knew the extent of spread of her disease and was never given an exact prognosis. So she has no way of knowing whether or not her profound transformation has in any way affected the course of her disease. However, as far as she is concerned her healing is complete now, and whether she dies sooner or later is completely irrelevent to her. This is an excellent example of the phenomenon of transformation. It perhaps also demonstrates the fact that it may be easier to 'let go' into this process if there isn't a lump confronting you by which you can continually gauge the completeness of your healing. It certainly also demonstrates that full-blown trans-formation can occur alongside full-blown medical treatment, thereby saving the patient agonising decisions about which 'camp' they are in.

## Dr Rees' views of the Centre's approach

Dr Rees is in favour of patients attending the Centre; in fact she has suggested it to some of her patients, but has had a mixed response. While some have found this helpful, others have been put off by the diet, or the distance to Bristol; yet others, she feels, have interpreted her suggestion as meaning that she had a lack of faith in the ability of the medical profession to give them further help, and have therefore imagined their condition was worse than it may have been. She thinks her advice may also be at odds with that of most local surgeons, many of whom feel that Bristol is a waste of time. She would always hope that patients would consider orthodox medical treatment as well as complementary therapy, but stresses that the final decision would be that of the patient.

Dr Rees is interested in the Centre's work, as she feels that orthodox medicine certainly does not have all the answers to cancer. However, she is sceptical about the use of vitamin and mineral therapy and she encourages patients to exercise dis-crimination in deciding which of the therapies are of relevance to them. Despite her views, she has never refused to prescribe the vitamins and has had no problem in doing this locally. She is in favour of counselling, healing and meditation but feels that visualisation is only useful to some people. She does believe that physical disease can be cured by the altering of emotional state and can therefore sees the obvious sense in trying to lift the patient mentally. However, she is also aware that any deterioration in mental state can have the reverse effect and is therefore very concerned that cancer patients are not given the opportunity to see themselves as failures, and that all counselling be done by highly experienced people, even in 'local support groups'.

Dr Rees points out that we will never know whether Evelyn's efforts have made any difference to the course of her disease as there is no tumour present to observe. She also thinks that there is probably no way in which the approach at Bristol can ever be assessed scientifically, as the programme is not suited to randomised controlled trials. She thinks, therefore, that we will probably never really know in concrete terms how valid is the Centre's approach. However, she says that her own attitude to cancer and the Centre were profoundly altered by another Centre patient who she looked after during her illness (before she met Evelyn). She was not only impressed by the lady's enthusiasm and commitment, but also by her amazing openness in discussing her disease, prognosis and death, and the obvious benefit she had derived from being counselled and sharing her burden amongst a group of caring individuals. This example was powerful enough to cause Dr Rees to review her own approach to the counselling of cancer patients.

She adds that if she had been Evelyn's GP at the time the diagnosis was made she would definitely have communicated her optimism to Evelyn. She says that in general she never lies to patients about their diagnoses, but tries to pick up signals from the patient about what they are ready to hear. She also takes into consideration what she thinks the patient's perception of cancer is and the likely consequences of their hearing the whole truth. She will then take whatever time she feels necessary to break the news in the way which will be the least devastating.

*Chapter 3*

# Joan Rowlatt
## Medical History
(*Birth Date*: 17 June 1914)

It has been a little difficult to get Joan's medical history or any comments on the Centre from her doctors because her GP retired just before I first went to see her and the new GP did not really feel in a position to discuss the personal aspects of her case. To complicate things still further she herself was in the process of moving from Gloucester to Oxford, so all her records were in transit between both GPs and consultants. Her original consultant did not feel he wanted to be involved anyway, as he said that he was unhappy about any of his patients being included in a series of retrospective case studies of an unproven form of therapy. He feels that the only way that advances are made is by prospective randomised studies. In fact he was never aware that when he was seeing her she was also attending Bristol. However, Joan reports that at their last consultation he was obviously surprised and delighted to see that Joan was still alive and well and he paid her the tribute that, "Whatever you are doing you should carry on, because you are obviously an expert in the management of your own disease".

I persisted anyway with Dr Parsons, her retired GP, who very kindly gave me the brief outline of her case. Joan had presented in April 1982 with a six month history of intermittent low abdominal pain and lethargy. She was referred to the surgeons, and on examination was found to have a palpable mass in her epigastrium. An exploratory laparotomy performed on 19.4.82 revealed the presence of a large tumour of the transverse colon; this was treated surgically with a hemicolectomy. Colostomy was not necessary. Histology of the excised material revealed the presence of extensive infiltrative adenocarcinoma. In April 1984 she was found to have a local recurrence of her tumour and was given a six weeks course of radiotherapy. She has been in clinical remission ever since.

Dr Parsons adds that, "It is certainly gratifying that this charming and gifted lady has survived so long, and there is no doubt of the tremendous psychological help she has derived from the Cancer Help Centre". However, he feels that it is utterly impossible to judge what effect her attendance at Bristol has had on the course of her disease as colonic tumours vary so widely in their rate of growth and metastasis. He does admit however, that no-one involved in the management of her case expected her to survive this long. On discovering that Joan was not just alive, but beaming, two months before they left for Oxford, he exclaimed to Mr Rowlatt, "Jack, it's nothing short of a miracle".

## Joan's Story

Joan has lived until recently on the most idyllic farm in the heart of Gloucestershire with her husband Jack. They have four children, all of whom are married, and nine grandchildren. Jack and Joan decided in 1985 that it was time they retired, and so in the summer of 1986 they sold their farm and moved to Oxfordshire, near the home of one of their daughters.

The first symptoms which Joan was aware of were psychological ones. Through the winter of 1981/1982 she felt depressed and edgy when she woke in the mornings, and generally debilitated mentally through her day. She feels that the onset was very insidious, and that these symptoms 'crept up on her' over a long period. The next development was of odd sensations in her tummy: at first she had isolated bouts of gut cramps which she just dismissed as indigestion. These attacks became more and more frequent. Her serious deterioration coincided with the beginning of lambing season in the spring of 1982. They had about two hundred ewes to lamb which meant being up around the clock for several days. Normally this was tiring but great fun. That year she just felt totally exhausted the whole time, but continually put off going to her doctor because she couldn't bring herself to leave her husband to cope alone. Neither Jack nor Joan had realised just how poorly she was until their daughter (who is a nurse) visited one day, and on seeing Joan immediately called the doctor. She had walked in just as

Joan was having a particularly bad pain, and was quite alarmed. She also thought her colour and general appearance appalling.

The doctor arrived and said that she needed to see a specialist, but feared it would take three months to get an opinion, because while she was ill, it could not be classed as an emergency, and she would have to go onto the waiting list. The family could not bear for Joan to have to wait like this, and they arranged for her to see the surgeon privately. It had not remotely occurred to Joan at this time that all this could be anything to do with cancer. She saw the surgeon three days later; he said, without hesitation, that he could feel a mass in her abdomen which he thought was a tumour. He wanted to operate immediately. Joan was very frightened; faced with this information and the NHS waiting lists the Rowlatts felt that they had no choice but to raise the money for private treatment so they found the £2000 for the operation. Their worst fears were confirmed when the tumour was diagnosed as being malignant. Despite the surgeon telling her the news after the operation, she has no recollection of this at all. She first 'heard' him say it on her return visit at six weeks. Her main feeling was one of complete bemusement and utter disbelief; it just didn't 'add up' for her and there was no way that she could even remotely contemplate dealing with this information.

The surgeon told her it would probably take about a year for her to recover from the operation as he had removed so much of the large bowel. In fact she says that she felt much better immediately after the operation although she can't be sure if this was just the relief of knowing it was out. When she asked him if she was going to recover completely, he replied rather hesitantly that he "thought so", but then added as he left the room, that he couldn't guarantee that there weren't any little bits left in her abdomen which might start to grow again. Joan immediately pushed this comment out of her mind thinking, "That's certainly not going to happen".

She was sixty-seven at the time of her operation so she didn't really expect to make the recovery of a young person. However she did get back into a passable state of health and returned to 'life as usual', until about two years later she found a lump on her tummy near her operation scar. She said it felt just like a baby's foot or arm feels when you're pregnant because sometimes it was there and sometimes it wasn't. She went to the GP who couldn't find it because of course it just wasn't there when she went to see him! He thought that the most likely explanation was that it was a small hernia in the scar and so reassured her. But she had a nasty nagging feeling that this wasn't right and eventually after seeing him a second time, went back to her surgeon. She was expecting or at least hoping for him to say just what the GP had said, and so she was shattered when he said that he couldn't find a hernia, and that "he thought it was the old enemy back".

He did not choose to operate again, presumably because he feared that the disease would be too widely disseminated within the abdomen and so he prescribed a six week course of radiation. The comment of the consultant was, "We've done really well so far, you've had two good years. We'll try and give you a bit longer with the radiotherapy". She was absolutely stunned by this comment because until that point, she still hadn't absorbed just how serious her illness was. She had never asked for, nor been given a prognosis and so had really stopped thinking of herself as ill. She had been living a busy active life since her operation and had been enjoying her family and her hobbies. not to mention her farm duties, so this was an absolute bolt out of the blue. She remembers feeling that it could not possibly be true. She says, "I knew it as a fact but I couldn't feel it — a bit like knowing there's something wrong with the car!"

The radiation made her incredibly ill. For six weeks she underwent sessions every weekday; she says at no stage during her illness had she felt as bad as she did during that treatment. She lost 28 pounds and felt weak, sick and lifeless. She had actually booked an appointment at Bristol just before going to see the consultant, and so had to cancel her appointment until her treatment was finished. She had a friend living locally who had derived great benefit from Bristol, and who, despite having introduced Joan to most of the ideas, felt that it would be much better for Joan to have first hand experience. After the radiotherapy had finished she was in such poor shape that her GP gently tried to dissuade her from going to Bristol, encouraging her to do what contemplative work she could at home. He very much gave her the impression that he thought she only had a matter of weeks to live. The other feeling he conveyed to her was that it was really pointless her trying to do anything about this herself, because it was 'bigger than her' and that it would be a waste of her time, money and effort. She should really use what precious little time she had left resting and being at home with her family.

She did come to Bristol however, and remembers vividly her first interview with Dr Greenwood. She was still very weak and ill from her radiotherapy and describes herself as being the colour of Horlick's malted milk. She was extremely demoralised by the GP's comments: while accepting the kindness of the spirit in which they were said, she still just could not believe that there was nothing she could do, that she must just accept that she was dying. Dr Greenwood asked her if she had anything to tell him and so she told him, with tears in her eyes, what the GP had said. He just took her by the hand and said, "Oh Joan, we just don't see it like that at all", and proceeded to explain all that she could still do for herself. She said it was absolute music to her ears and she could feel the relief flooding through her. She says, "That moment was so wonderful that it is impossible to describe". It was her turning point. From that moment on she voraciously took up and practised absolutely everything which was suggested to her. She carried on through that day getting happier and happier. She says, "I was so uplifted. I didn't think I could be that uplifted by anything or anybody. It wasn't just the doctor, it was everything. What people said, the attitudes, and the love — it was just incredible — I don't think I could ever put it into words. I just knew deep inside myself that somehow I was going to cope."

Her friend, Jill Tonner, had prepared Joan very well, and had said to her that she was already half way there as she was so receptive. So Joan had gone really well primed and expecting to receive help, but actually when she got home she rang Jill and said, "Even you couldn't describe how wonderful it was". It had surpassed all her expectations. She remembers thinking, "Why can't everybody with cancer come here", but she now fully acknowledges that it just isn't for everybody.

The diet was very hard for Joan and her family to follow initially because they were in her words "typical farmers — meat and two veg with plenty of fresh eggs, butter, cream, and cheese". So she made the changeover very gradually. Jack became a real hero with the organic carrots, scrubbing a bucket-full for her every day for her carrot juice. She feels intuitively that the diet has probably been the cornerstone of her recovery and wonders if this is because her cancer was abdominal, thinking either that the diet has affected her gut directly in a nourishing and healing way or that maybe previously she was eating something that was carcinogenic. She has a sneaking feeling it might be as simple as that. For this reason she has never relaxed the diet, despite having been nervous at first because of the high fibre content. She says that having a disease of the gut makes you extremely insecure anyway. It is your core, and, as such, affects every part of you. (Joan says she could have handled having the cancer in a limb or breast far more easily.) As with many of the Centre's gut cancer patients she now swears by the diet. Even those with colostomies and ileostomies often find, after an initial readjustment period, that all works more smoothly than ever. She also has great faith in the vitamin and mineral supplementation and has continued to take her full quota.

The counselling was extremely helpful to Joan. She had a very difficult childhood; her parents were very unhappily married and their respective families were in a state of constant feud. She was the fourth of five children and Joan feels that her mother grew to dislike her over the years because she was "the image of my father's family" — auburn and artistic. Her mother didn't physically abuse her, but there was a constant torrent of verbal abuse. She would tell Joan over and over again that she was hopeless and that no one would ever love her. This caused Joan to be in a state of severe emotional stress all her life and not surprisingly, she was left with an appalling self image. She felt good about her father but he was rather a remote figure and she was afraid to show him affection for fear of incurring yet more of her mother's wrath. Every now and then they would share odd moments alone and he would be very sweet to her. This would always make her cry — she could hardly bear it. Up until very recently Joan continued to have nightmares about her mother.

Anthony Elman, one of the Centre's counsellors, helped her greatly with this. He got her to talk to and comfort her 'child' and to get the child to write down every way in which her mother hurt her. Having done this she was to tear up the piece of paper and throw it away. He then did a visualisation with her where he got her to bring her wounded child and her shadowy cancer into her mind's eye simultaneously and then asked her to pour healing light and love over them both. The nightmare never recurred after that session and Joan remembers it with enormous gratitude as an experience both profound and help-ful. Later he worked with her on understanding and forgiving her mother.

A further area of difficulty for Joan has been her home situation. Joan and her husband are as different as chalk and cheese. They adore and have utmost respect for each other, but really have very little in common. Jack is a completely down to earth, practical, unemotional, non-verbal man of the earth, while Joan, on the other hand, is like quicksilver — highly sensitive, artistic, imaginative, and emotional, with a great need for self-expression and articulation of her thoughts and feelings. They met at the Stratford Mop one year. Joan fell off a round-about and Jack caught her!

It would never occur to you from Jack's appearance that he could be anything other than a farmer, whereas to look at Joan you would think her anything other than a farmer's wife. One would probably place her as a teacher or artist, certainly as a person of words and music. To be as sensitive as she, and to have spent her whole life in the farming environment has meant that she has been rather like a sea anemone with all it's tentacles curled up all the time. Her way of coping, as during her childhood, was to hide her feelings in order to maintain peace. Always, she would do anything to avoid the possibility of rejection, and this included suppressing any anger that she might feel. She feels that it is not only her emotional sensitivity that she has kept hidden away, but also her spiritual sensitivity, and that at last the door to her spiritual garden is finally open. The recognition of her true nature by the people at the Centre, even at this late stage in her life, has been deeply liberating for her. Of course, her guilt and uneasiness go back to her mother's dismissal of Joan as a child. So, like Evelyn, her real healing has come about through being validated as a person. She, too, has finally shed the guilt she feels for being alive, and now finally feels accepted into the human race.

She had thrown herself fully into her role as 'farmer's wife' but she will admit that it has always required that bit of a push. Her acceptance was due to the fact that it just wasn't in her repertoire to ask for what she wanted. She felt she just had to keep on proving her worthiness. This doesn't mean that if she had her time again she would necessarily do anything differ-

ently. One thing she is enormously content with is how different
an experience she created for her children from that of her own
childhood. She is aware though, that there is a part of herself
that she has always 'sold short'. As with Evelyn, through the
experience of her illness and healing she is now far more
contented, and is less resistant to her husband's ways. As a
result their relationship has become far warmer and deeper. Of
course the other side of the coin is that the threat to her life has
caused Jack to take her presence far less for granted and so they
are generally much more attentive to each other, and Jack has
finally become able to verbalise his great love for, and need of,
Joan.

Another aspect of her counselling which was very helpful to
Joan was that she undertook a 'guided dying' meditation with
one of her counsellors. In Joan's case it wasn't so much her fear
of dying that was the problem but more her sense of bewilderment and non-acceptance of death as a possibility. At the point
at which death seemed quite imminent, it was considered a good
idea consciously to rehearse her approach to dying so that she
would be a little calmer when the time came. She felt this to be
of tremendous benefit, because, when actually confronted with
the scenario, she found herself able to cope. One of the main
aspects of her difficulty, she discovered, was her fear of causing
pain and hurt to others by dying. The counsellor was able to
help her confront and begin to shed this terrible burden. She had
spent all her life needing to keep up a constant surveillance of
the needs of others which then of course would always get
complete priority. This breakthrough greatly enabled her to
voice her own needs. She chuckles as she says, "My husband
was astounded!"

Joan needed little encouragement to set her creativity going
but paradoxically her piano playing fell off once she had started
to recover; she had always played her piano every day during
her entire adult life, if only for ten minutes. It was her
sanctuary. Fascinatingly, as she began to open up and bring the
hidden part of herself out of the shadows, she no longer felt the
need for her piano and sold it. This has actually been an
unexpected release to her. She has also always found great
solace in painting and this she has not given up. One of her
major pleasures is painting meadow flowers in the Spring and
Summer. She says that when she sees such natural beauty in the

fields she feels the beauty inside herself as a healing force. She constantly sees things she looks at as pictures. In fact she said that she was "painting you in my mind's eye" the whole time we were talking. An extraordinary thing happens when Joan starts to paint: she does not feel that it is her doing the painting — it's just suddenly all there on the canvas to her complete amazement.

She regularly takes a half hour quiet time in her day to relax and meditate. She uses tape recordings to help her do this. She enjoys Ludi How's tape (from the Centre) which is primarily an imaging tape, directed at stimulating right-brain activity. She also has some tapes of a Reverend Jack Burton who was once a minister but has now left the church to practise healing full time. In his tapes he tends to take a thought from Christian scripture and expand it, but not in a preaching fashion, she hastens to add. She finds concentrating on his words and the feeling that emanates from him most relaxing.

She describes herself as being a "bit poor at imaging" and then in the next breath told me of her wonderful success at using imaging to protect her skin during radiotherapy. The technicians told her that she would suffer burns on her back from the radiation. They asked her to tell them when this started to happen so that they could alter the direction of the radiation. On one of Dr Alec Forbes' tapes she'd heard of a person who'd had to have radiotherapy through the roof of his mouth. This used to burn terribly until he learnt how to image. His technique was to image that the only place the rays could touch was the cancer. In her treatment sessions she was given four thirty-second bursts of radiation. She thought that she could just about concentrate for this long. So every time she heard the click of the machine she would concentrate intensely on the fact that the only place that the rays could touch was her cancer. She was completely successful — she had no skin marking at all. Apparently the staff of the radiotherapy unit were absolutely amazed. She certainly finds it impossible to do the Simonton type of imaging as she can't bear aggression of any sort — doubtless a legacy from her childhood.

Another successful use of imaging she has made has been to protect herself during the stress of moving house, using an image that was given to her by Barbara Siddall, a counsellor at the Centre. Barbara had anticipated that Joan's move out of the farm, where she and her family had lived for the previous twenty years, could be highly traumatic, both practically and emotionally. Her suggestion to Joan was that she imagined herself to be in a big see-through bubble with a very tough skin. That way she could see everything that was going on but none of it would have to impinge on her — she could just float through it. Joan found this invaluable and in fact was the strong one who got everybody else through the move!

Joan goes into positive raptures about her experience of healing. It gives her a sense of deep relaxation and receptivity in which she is open to healing energy. In this state she feels an actual physical sensation of a glowing strength entering her. Initially she had healing from a man who lived locally who was a spiritualist. When he moved away from the area she went to a local minister, and would sometimes receive healing from three people simultaneously in a healing circle. Although there were qualities to these healings which were subtly different, she had this same strengthening feeling from both experiences. More recently, when she was praising and thanking the group for their help, they said "It's actually you that gives us healing and inspiration". I have heard this so many times that I begin to wonder if, for some people their dis-ease is actually their having no outlet for the enormous amount of love which they have to give. In a healing situation, rather like in electrical circuits, the 'current' will flow in the direction of the greatest gradient. So, in these situations it could be possible that what makes the 'patient' feel better is the allowing of some of this loving energy to be released.

She has had a session with one of the Centre's healers, however, which "did very little for her" and so she too would urge people to keep searching until they find the right healer for them. Despite having been involved in the Church for years, she says she has never experienced the spiritual uplift she received through healing and through her visits to the Centre. She had been very involved with Christian Science, but when she became ill she actually found their approach rather less helpful than Bristol's because she feels that they go too far in terms of ignoring the body. She feels that while much of the Christian Science philosophy is sound and prepared her well for Bristol, there is too much denial of the earthly and material realities. One of her more unusual sources of healing has been her cat!

Joan would spend hours while she was ill cuddling, stroking and loving her cat, finding that this too would allow her to wind down and get into the receptive healing state.

One of the unexpected benefits of her attendance at Bristol has been the effect that the approach and the philosophy has had on her family. Apparently all of her children vie to take her to Bristol and that includes her two sons, one a policeman, the other a farmer. They sit around talking the ideas over and over; several family members now eat the Bristol diet and all have been involved, one way or another, in fund raising and support of the Centre. She overflows with praise of them all for the way they have looked after her: she feels that it was almost worse for them than for her — especially for Jack. She says that they weren't overly fussy, just practically and solidly behind her. The effects of her trips to Bristol are "like ripples on a pond", she says, "which just keep spreading and spreading. Sometimes," she adds, "I could just burst with gratitude."

Despite all the positive feelings she has about self-help, Joan would still go back to the medical profession for help if she got further symptoms. She definitely does not feel there has to be a choice between orthodox and complementary medicine and expresses extreme gratitude for the medical treatment she has received. Her comment to the medical profession would be that she wishes "everyone could be gentler with you". She feels strongly that either the pressure of work, emotional discomfort or general over-exposure of doctors to horrific situations makes them very poor at empathising with the patient's difficulties. She can understand this more with the hospital based doctors, considering the pressures that they are under to keep the conveyor belt rolling along, but thinks that GP's should spend far more time in the counselling and educational roles than they do presently. She feels they should also be far more careful in assessing who it is they are dealing with. She is the type of person who doesn't want to know the gory details as she is such a visual person that the images haunt her. One doctor said to her that she shouldn't worry, there was plenty of room inside for the tumours to grow before they hit a vital spot! This comment alone gave her nightmares for weeks. She is also the kind of person who only wants the questions she asks answered and doesn't want to know the rest. Of course there are other patients who throw their hands up in horror saying 'the doctor never told me anything!' The skill is obviously in judging which is which and in treating each individual appropriately.

Joan's story again illustrates that transformation and full medical treatment can go hand in hand. It also illustrates the fact that it is never too late to grasp life with both hands, either in terms of one's age or the stage of the disease. When I saw Joan, despite the fact that her home was being dismantled all around her, she was brimming over with life and enthusiasm. I came away feeling positively refreshed and very privileged to have met her.

## Chapter 4

# Katherina Collins

## Medical History

(*Birth Date*: 14 July 1932)

*Supplied by Katherina's GP, Dr Douglas Latto, with additional information from the Florida Medical Centre, Lauderdale Lakes, Florida.*

A small breast lump was first noticed by Katherina circa 1971. Its growth was greatly accelerated after the death of her husband in 1973 and the tumour broke the skin in the summer of that year. Katherina failed to present to her GP, Dr Douglas Latto until July 1st, 1981. He made an immediate clinical diagnosis of fungating cancer of the breast. He referred her to the Guy's hospital breast unit, but she did not attend. He then tried to get Katherina to see his brother Conrad who is a surgeon, but she would not do this either. That summer she went to stay with her family in America and finally, under heavy pressure from them, had a lumpectomy at the Florida Medical Centre.

Their diagnosis was that of Fungating Ductal Carcinoma of the left breast. The histology report read as follows:-

a. Extensive dermal infiltration by ductal carcinoma,

b. Extensive residual infiltrating ductal carcinoma at the biopsy site and

c. seven out of seven positive axillary lymph nodes.

Bone and liver scans were performed and found to be normal. She was then given the prognosis that if she underwent a mastectomy, radio- and chemotherapy she may have a life expectancy of around two years. With no treatment she could only expect to live about four to six months or until around Christmas of 1981. Despite the gloomy prognosis Katherina did not have a mastectomy or any of the other treatment suggested. She returned home to England and by October 27th, 1981 when she saw Dr Latto again, was found to have already developed a large local recurrence in the same breast. This was confirmed by Mr Conrad Latto. Katherina still refused to have the further surgery which was urgently recommended by him.

At this point Dr Latto accepted that Katherina would not accept any medical treatment and decided to support her in any alternative treatment she may decide to try, which included her attendance at the Bristol Cancer Help Centre. He encouraged her to eat a strict low protein diet and was happy to give her Iscador and B12 injections. Katherina has had no other medical treatment for her breast lump since her lumpectomy in the U.S.

Dr Latto continued to see Katherina regularly and to his delight was able to inform Katherina that as the weeks went by the lump was getting smaller and that the skin was healing. In 1983 she was declared clinically clear by both Dr Douglas Latto and Mr Conrad Latto. Dr Latto's own words when talking to me were that, "My brother and I watched the tumour disappear before our very eyes!" She has had no local or distant recurrence since this time.

**Author's Comment**. Ductal carcinoma is a relatively non-aggressive type of cancer of the breast as compared with the more common adenocarcinoma. It is for this reason that Katherina was able to cope for such a long period before attending her GP. In general terms this approach is not recommended and any person discovering unusual lumps is advised to attend their GP immediately. Once a diagnosis is made an individual may then decide in an informed manner how to deal with her situation. The comparative benignity of ductal carcinoma is due to the fact that lymph nodes become involved late in the course of the disease. However, due to Katherina's failure to present to her doctor for some years after first being aware of her lump, her disease had already progressed to the life threatening stage (as reflected in the prognosis given to her in America). Katherina's recovery is therefore highly unusual in medical terms and is a wonderful example of the application of holistic principles as will be seen from reading her story. However had she presented to her GP earlier, in her particular case the disease need never have reached the life threatening stage.

## Katherina's Story

Katherina was born on the 14th July, 1932 in London. She describes herself as having been incredibly lucky to have had such a beautiful family and such a happy early life. Her parents both came from Georgia, Russia, but they met in London and married here. She describes them as wonderful people who were extremely open minded and unprejudiced. She is the youngest of five children and has two brothers and two sisters. She married her husband Gabriel in London. He was 29 years older than she and was like a father as well as a husband to her. She loved him very dearly and they had an extremely happy close marriage which produced two sons, Jack and Harry. Her husband ran a business in London and Katherina both helped him in his business and was involved in a business of her own within the fashion world. One of Katherina's brothers, Sam, who is an artist, moved to the United States thirty years ago, while her other brother and sisters stayed in and around London and they have all remained very close to each other. Many members of her mother's family also moved to America, where several of their children were to become doctors.

In 1964 Gabriel became seriously ill with what was later diagnosed to be cancer of the stomach. His illness lasted nine years during which time Katherina was constantly at his side. They received tremendous support through this period from Dr Latto who became a close friend.

Katherina says that Gabi was incredibly sweet natured and hardly ever complained during the whole gruelling nine years, during the early part of which Katherina was not told the true diagnosis. She eventually discovered accidentally when one of the nurses, assuming Katherina knew, offered her condolences. Once the information was out of the bag the doctors in charge strongly advised Katherina not to tell her husband saying it would kill him if he knew. She was beside herself with worry and grief and her memory of that period is very dim and hazy now. She says that if she'd allowed herself to feel the pain it would have killed her; she cannot imagine how she got through living out this dreadful charade with her husband, continually reassuring him and playing games with him in an attempt to keep him from realising just how ill he was or from naming the disease. She even bought him identical clothes to those he already had at home, but in smaller sizes so that he wouldn't realise how much weight he'd lost. He eventually died in 1973 having been intravenously fed for a whole year. Katherina now feels strongly that he should have been told that he had cancer so that they could have shared their pain and fears.

Katherina first noticed the lump in her breast during this terrible ordeal with her husband. She had strong suspicions that the lump was cancerous right from the very moment she discovered it but her emotional burdens were far too great to cope with confirmation of this diagnosis. Her own needs, she felt, were secondary to those of her husband. It was a full time job looking after him, her children and the business — how could she possibly be ill herself? Neither could she bear the thought of worrying her family with a second cancer, so she didn't confide in anyone; her reaction was to push it to the back of her mind, which was not too difficult as it didn't seem to be growing and wasn't painful.

However she was to receive yet another catastrophic blow. Within five weeks of her husband's death the bailiffs arrived and took all their possessions and property, including their house. Tragically their business had not been insured and all their personal belongings were taken in lieu of debts incurred during the long illness. Katherina and the two boys (now aged nineteen and fifteen) were rehoused in a one bedroomed council flat. This was the point at which her cancer 'really broke'. The lump started to grow rapidly, actually breaking through the skin within two or three weeks of this second calamity. She remembers feeling so utterly despondent at this time; that she no longer cared if the disease spread right through her, or even whether she lived or died. All her plans were shattered, she felt there could be no future at all and she had nothing left with which to support her sons and thought she was now useless to them. She had lost her husband and felt she could no longer fulfil her role as mother. There was nothing left and death appeared to be "a good way out".

For the next seven years she watched her cancer grow, only finally approaching her old friend and GP Douglas Latto when her pain and fear became unbearable. When he asked why she had come she told him outright that she had cancer. While she knew this with one part of mind she was really trying to goad him into telling her that that was nonsense. He did say something along these lines until she got undressed, at which point his face revealed all and her game of denial was abruptly over. He could not conceal his shock and upset at the sight of her raw tumour. Having recollected himself he tried very hard to make as light as he could of the situation, reassuring Katherina that she would be admitted very quickly to hospital to have the breast removed and that all would then be well. He genuinely wanted to make things as easy as possible for her, knowing only too well of the living nightmare of the previous years. Katherina could see that he was horrified at the extent of the tumour and she too was devastated by this confirmation of her worst fears. Remembering that day she says, "I just thought he'd say, 'Of course you haven't got cancer you silly date' — and there was I, having said for the previous years that I didn't care if I lived or died and now suddenly, oh boy, did I care?"

She is still amazed at just how strong the urge to cling to life was at that moment despite the fact that her whole world appeared to be in ruins. When asked what she thought was at the root of this feeling she answered that she is sure that it was the fear of death. She feels that while many cancer patients state that what is hardest for them is the fear of pain, or their sadness at the thought of not being able to do all those things they had planned to do, what really unites them all is the terror of death. She feels that to most people the diagnosis of cancer is a death sentence and that no one who hasn't been sentenced to death can even begin to imagine how it makes you feel; the lack of comprehension of this state by others causes or allows you to sink very deeply inside yourself. It is as if you know you are dying anyway, so nothing anyone says makes any real difference. It is impossible for them to reach you. All the positive things people may say you can see as being very sweet and well intentioned but are never the less powerless against the *knowledge* that you are going to die. This understanding gave her new insight into her husband's state of mind once it had become obvious that he was never going to get better. She says that although she had imagined that she had been aware of his every thought she now realises that she hadn't had a clue. The extent of her fear really surprised Katherina because, as a medium who has contact with the spiritual plane, she has a firm belief in life after death and so had always considered herself to have no fear of dying. But such was her fear at times during this period that she was actually afraid to sleep at night fearing that death might follow if her concentration lapsed for even one minute.

The timing of the diagnosis coincided with a visit from the United States by her brother Sam. Katherina plucked up the courage to tell him and then to tell her sons. His immediate reaction was to invite her to return with him to the States. She can clearly remember thinking that it would suit her fine to go back there with him and be cared for while she died. She agreed to go, on condition that he would not force her to have any medical treatment, although she did promise that she would speak to one of her doctor cousins. She says that the flight to America was horrific. Sam and Katherina didn't know what to say to each other and her sister-in-law was equally at a loss when they arrived. She put off meeting her cousin and also took a long time to get round to see the specialist that he had recommended when she did eventually see him. She knew perfectly well that all they could offer her was an operation, because Dr Latto had told her that. She had always used natural therapies herself, but does not think that this was at the root of her resistance to medical treatment. She traces it mainly to the growing distrust of the medical profession that she had accumulated during her husband's illness. She had seen the doctors cause as many problems as they had solved, had abhorred that process which reduced her husband to a heap of skin and bones, dependent for life on drips, catheters, suction pumps and drugs. Her other thought was that if she were to become that ill who would look after her? He'd had her to run back and forth to the hospital three times a day but who did she have? This was not self-pity, it was reality. Unable to bear the thought of being that kind of burden to anybody else, she was quite determined to stay out of hospital.

However at this stage, pressure on her began to mount. The specialist was adamant that she needed treatment, and so her brother invited Harry, her youngest son, to come to America to see whether he could persuade Katherina to accept treatment for his sake. The consultant even tried to use scare tactics, giving her a graphic description of exactly what was likely to happen to her as the secondaries really took hold. He told her to stop being so incredibly stupid and to have an urgent mastectomy. She said that she "needed time to think about it", to which he replied that she had no time left for thinking. While the doctor continued to discuss the prognosis with others present, Katherina dressed, and completely unobserved, left the hospital.

Under enormous pressure from her family over the next few weeks she finally agreed to have a lumpectomy and biopsy of nearby lymph nodes and scans to assess the extent of secondaries. The diagnosis of malignancy was then finally made and, what was worse, the tumour had now spread to seven out of seven lymph nodes biopsied. The scan had not, however, revealed distant spread of the cancer. The surgeon wanted to go on to perform more radical surgery, extensive radiotherapy and to instigate chemotherapy immediately, knowing from the biopsy report that he had not cleared all the cancerous cells with the first operation. Katherina dug her heels in, firmly refusing any other medical treatment. She was told by the surgeon that with treatment her prognosis was around two years, without, she might not survive until Christmas of that year, a mere four months away. She could have stayed on in the United States but felt she was just waiting there to die. This placed an unbearable strain on all involved in the light of her refusal to accept treatment. She decided to come home.

Within just four weeks of her return the lump had grown back, but was now twice its previous size. She went again to Dr Latto who referred her to his brother, Mr Conrad Latto, once more. He, too, was keen to perform a mastectomy. Katherina again declined. At this point she and Dr Latto confronted the fact that they were at an impasse regarding medical treatment, and he agreed to support her in any other way that he could. In addition to this attitude, acknowledged a tremendous help by Katherina, he also started to explore some alternative avenues. His first discovery was of the anthroposophical treatment Iscador. She started and has never stopped having weekly injections of Iscador. She firmly believes in its benefits, saying that she feels better after its injection.

Now one of the hardest things was to cope with the reaction of her family in England. Katherina feels that those close to the cancer patient most commonly react in one of two ways: they either smother the person with 'sickly' love and affection or otherwise distance themseves. Both types of reaction arise from the fact that they cannot bear the thought that the person whom they love may soon be gone. What made things much more difficult for Katherina's family was that she seemed to be on an active suicide mission because she was refusing medical treatment. This not surprisingly caused them to feel completely frustrated and impotent, which in turn caused Katherina to retreat still further into her obstinate stance. It appears that paradoxically their reaction may have been Katherina's saving grace. Up to this point, although she was quite sure how she felt about the medical treatment, she had no alternative in mind and did not believe she was going to make it. Somehow her family's lack of ability to understand the way she had to deal with her illness caused her to become determined to prove to them that she could do it her way. She says, "That was the turning point which saved my life — I was angry enough to want to live".

She was now on the verge of an enormous and challenging journey of self-discovery. Now that she had decided to live she had to find the way to rid herself of her disease; it was as if she had entered a state of deep self-sufficiency. She knew that it was completely up to her, and what is more in this new state she knew that somewhere inside herself she had the knowledge necessary to cure her cancer. She is dubious as to whether any therapist could have brought her to this point. It was the intensity of the emotions aroused in her by her struggle with her family which brought her to this very profound state of self-confrontation.

She started investigating the world of alternative cancer treatment. She was hoping to find help in this process of unearthing her self-healing potential. However, before getting any help she had a very interesting insight: she realised that during her husband's illness she had somehow put the cancer 'on hold'. What had changed the course of the disease and allowed the cancer to grow following Gabi's death had been a change in her mental and emotional state. Once her husband had died, and her material possessions had gone, she had felt utterly valueless — as if there was no point to her life. Once locked into this frame of mind her cancer had grown quickly. She now knew that somehow she had to get back into the state of mind that she had been in whilst nursing her husband. The first big hurdle had been crossed — she really wanted to live. The next major step forward she realised would be to learn to love, nourish and value herself in the way she had valued her husband; to feel as valued and validated in the task of resurrecting and nursing herself as she had done in the task of nursing him.

After addressing herself to her mental attitude the area Katherina came upon next was diet. Although having always been a vegetarian she drank a lot of tea and coffee and smoked cigarettes. Instinctively she felt that she must completely clean out her body, and immediately gave up these habits. She then put herself on a grape fast, having found a book describing this approach in the cancer section of her local library. This involved her in eating nothing other than four pounds of grapes each day, which she did for around eight weeks, feeling the benefit very quickly. The most significant factor obviously was that her tumour stopped growing, but she also says that her whole body began to feel different — far lighter and less clogged. Her fingernails got stronger and so did her hair (actually beginning to curl for the first time in her life!). This was all tremendously encouraging to her. She had proved to herself that she could exert some control over her bodily processes.

At this time the tumour was still very large and raw, and the pain was unbearable. This was a great problem for Katherina as both her lifelong philosophy and her diet prevented her from taking any drugs. Again using her intuition she hit upon the idea of an exercise bicycle and hand grips. Whenever she was in pain she would distract herself and kill the pain at the same time by peddling furiously on her bicycle or squeezing hard on the hand grips. (Not long after her discovery, work was published about the connection between exercise and the release of pain-killing endorphins in the brain!) It was now eighteen months since her diagnosis in the United States, and she was still alive and had managed to stop her tumour from growing.

It was at this point that she first learned about the existence of the Bristol Cancer Help Centre. Listening to the radio one day she heard the Centre being discussed. Her feeling of relief was enormous, having felt totally isolated in what, to her friends and family, was a completely lunatic approach to her disease. She arrived at the Centre in May 1982, still extremely ill and looking very weak indeed by all reports. The most potent part of this first visit for Katherina was what she describes as, "such genuine love from strangers". There was real affection and plenty of hugs and cuddles from people who weren't afraid of her or her cancer. This unexpected warmth gradually began to melt away her wall of isolation. She explored all the different forms of therapy that the Centre offered. Whilst acknowledging the value and importance of all of them she does not attach any special significance to any one of them; rather believing that all the therapists who treated her helped to consolidate her belief in her own power and the notion that she could be well again. She felt that the subtle internal adjustments which then had to be made were entirely up to her. Nobody could really sense her state better than she and certainly nobody else could make the necessary changes.

The Centre provided the fuel in the form of love and encouragement to keep Katherina on her journey of self-discovery. She goes so far as to say that she probably would not be here now if not for the Centre. Although she was 'on the right track' she doesn't know how long she could have sustained her efforts and faith in isolation. The Centre provided a haven for her and a feeling of 'being held', which allowed her to relax and stop the searching for a cure, instead being stiller and looking inside herself for the answers. She feels that many people who come to the Centre do so still in the spirit of searching for a cure or "magic bullet" and so go away feeling disappointed or empty handed. In this search for a cure outside themselves she believes them to be wasting precious time and energy that they could be directing towards the real issue of being well!

Miraculously over the next year Katherina's tumour shrank until it finally disappeared. Her GP pronounced her clinically clear in 1983. She is now fully returned to her normal health and vigour and is quite radiant. She exudes a quiet sense of discipline, wisdom and self-knowledge, balanced by a delightful sense of humour and great warmth. She has gone from strength to strength and is now totally dedicated to the helping of other cancer patients. To this end she now runs a highly valued support group in East London. Whilst believing that the controlling of the disease is ultimately an entirely personal matter she does this work because she never wants any cancer patient anywhere to feel isolated again. She acknowledges the paradox in this because for her it was through reaching that very point of feeling completely abandoned, reaching her very lowest ebb, that she came to the turning point in her illness.

Whilst I was talking to Katherina her telephone rang and she suddenly switched roles into that of counsellor. At the other end of the line was a distraught woman with cancer who had heard about Katherina's group. The warmth and compassion which flowed down that telephone line was quite extraordinary and very moving. The caller, despite living with her husband and family was describing exactly the agonising isolation Katherina had been trying to explain to me moments before. Katherina outlined to her the many ways in which the group could offer support and most importantly of all, that now she had made contact she need never feel alone again; every single person in the group had been through exactly what she was going through now, there was no need for her to feel silly or embarrassed. Members of the group could give her healing and counselling, practical help regarding diet, and of course there would always be hugs, reassurance and lots of encouragement. It was possible to fight and even cure cancer. I could almost feel the woman relax in the warmth of Katherina's great presence and love.

In addition to the work she does with the support group, she also spends one and a half days a week at the Centre, encouraging other patients. She is so involved in this work that she sometimes feels that she could do it seven days a week, and says that is because she is in a hurry for everyone to realise just what this sort of approach is all about. Whilst knowing that this is out of the question as far as her own health is concerned, she still finds it frustrating to know that for every patient who has begun to think holistically about their cancer there are hundreds who haven't ever heard of these ideas.

## Katherina's healing

Katherina has found, by trial and error, her way of regaining and maintaining her health. She is a firm believer in the importance of diet. She still sticks closely to the Bristol diet, eating significantly more raw food than she used to whilst on her former vegetarian diet. She maintains that the physical benefits of the diet are obvious, essential and beyond question. What is equally important to her is the benefit of the mental discipline involved in keeping to the diet. She feels that this is one of the only outward signs of her intention to be well and feels that the discipline involved in remaining on the diet strengthens her resolve to keep the other, even more slippery,

parts of her being in order! It serves as a daily reminder that you
intend to nurture yourself in an entirely different way. She
therefore disagrees with the practice at Bristol of relaxing the
diet after three months as she feels this facilitates the process of
falling back into other subtle self-destructive behaviour patterns
and attitudes. If ever she is ill one of her major treatments is still
to go on a grape fast as she feels this is one of the quickest ways
to disperse symptoms. She has tailored her intake of vitamins
and minerals to what she intuitively believes to be right for her.
She has great faith in vitamin C and still takes 12 to 14 grams
daily, along with Selenium and Zinc. She makes fresh carrot
juice daily as she believes this is the far superior way of taking
vitamin A, and, as mentioned above, still has weekly injections
of Iscador.

Spiritual healing is important to Katherina. She has healing at
the Centre from Christopher Pilkington and also from the
healers who come to her support group. She describes feeling
sensations of both heat and cold which 'come through' on
different occasions. She has never had a spectacular healing. If
she goes in with a pain she comes out with a pain, but she
always feels better. She finds the experience relaxing at a far
deeper level than physical relaxation. Another way she would
describe this is as a spiritual uplift "It is as if someone has come
along and taken off the internal pressure of the anxiety and
fear". To get this lift she feels she has to be in tune with her
healer: in the past she has received healing from someone whom
she didn't 'feel good about', which resulted in her feeling
physically sick. (This she sees as another example of her
instincts telling her what is beneficial for her.) Unfortunately on
that occasion she didn't follow her feelings, but it has been
similar experiences which have helped her to learn to trust and
develop her instincts. When 'in tune' with her healer she often
finds that her own psychic faculty is more pronounced which
can be of benefit not only to her but also to the healer, as if a
state of reciprocal healing is achieved. In this state she often
feels the presence of a spiritual guide and healer.

Katherina attempts to do some relaxation and meditation
daily, finding relaxation easier after exerting herself physically.
She meditates sitting upright in a chair, allowing her mind to 'go
completely blank'. Initially she had great problems with this
because she was such a worrier; her mind would jump around

from one problem to another. When this happenened she would determinedly start the process again until she got it right. She can now achieve quite a profound state of meditation in which she is totally present, completely awake and aware, but her mind is empty. This leaves her with a great sense of well-being.

However, the most impressive and potent source of her self-help is her mental attitude and mind control. I feel this is her real magic. She seems to have worked out the relationship between her exact state of mind and her physical body and has learnt to identify moods, feelings, attitudes and thought patterns which drag her down physically. Now when these occur she consciously (often through a great act of will) shifts her attention to 'non-toxic' mental material. This may sound easy, but try to imagine even once letting go of feelings of self-pity, loneliness, anger and fear! For Katherina the time has passed when she could wait for or rely on others to come to her emotional rescue. We are most of us far too self-indulgent to even imagine doing this.

Occasionally when her control slips and odd symptoms occur she can actually cause them to disappear by use of this technique. For example when she had lymphoedema (swelling) of her legs and was told that this may be due to a recurrence of her cancer, she had actually caused the symptom to disappear by the time she had completed her bus ride home! From her refusal even to acknowledge the possibility that there is any cancer in her body it therefore follows that there just could not be a symptom which could be associated with cancer. She deliberately avoids talking about (or even knowing where the organs in her body are) where secondaries would be likely to occur. This is so that she never focuses any fear on them, convinced that so doing makes the possibility of cancer growing there more likely. She never thinks of herself as ill. During the time between her attitude change and the disappearance of her tumour she wouldn't even look at her breast for these same reasons, and so only discovered the tumour had gone when Dr Latto told her!

She feels that another problem for the cancer sufferer is that, not only do they imagine that every ache or pain is due to a re-emergence of the disease, but that all the health care professionals think in this way too; this collusive atmosphere, she says, brings about the perfect environment for a tumour to grow. For this reason she tries to avoid practitioners of any sort as she feels that even holistic practitioners fall into this trap. Katherina also uses her mental discipline to control her perception of pain — she simply does not allow herself to feel it because, she says, every pain becomes cancer, and if that happens you might as well "put yourself in bed and forget it". She always keeps herself "up, out and doing." This sort of practice could of course be called a very elaborate denial mechanism. Usually the practice of denial is regarded pretty suspiciously by psychotherapists and medical practitioners. Katherina's use of this mechanism certainly highlights the possibility of the difference between using it to hide from the truth and using it to change the 'truth'. The impressive results which she has now achieved certainly demand the study of the positive sides of this denial technique. Her level of mind control and self-discipline is reminiscent of high yogic practice, which she has again stumbled upon through intuition, because of her complete determination to live.

Katherina now feels a lot more comfortable with the thought of death. She says, "At the beginning it was all death and nothing else — all I could see was death. I was scared to go out or go to sleep in case I dropped dead. Because I was alone it was worse. I was completely shut down. There was nothing psychic about me in those first few months after diagnosis. I couldn't give myself any space, it was just me and me and me." She feels it's as if there is a breaking point. "You either have to rid yourself of the fear or the fear itself will kill you, never mind the cancer! You just can't keep that much fear inside you." She gradually began to see that she was wasting what precious little time she had, because while she was so fearful she was not living at all. So, little by little, as she re-embraced life her fear began to fade. She now feels that the fear is almost completely gone although she does occasionally have short lapses back into the loneliness of the cancer patient. Fortunately these negative feelings are quickly alleviated by her trips into the Centre or to her own group.

Her attitude towards herself shifted the day she decided she was angry enough to live. At that point she learned that she valued herself just for being her, not as a wife or as a mother or as a business woman. From having sunk to the bottom of a pit of despair, self-pity and loneliness, she fought her way back, steadily rebuilding her self image and is now a source of strength and inspiration to many. The extent to which this has been an internal process for Katherina is reflected by the fact that her notes at the Centre are only two pages long. It is a real paradox to sit with her thin file and hear the Katherina say how much she has gained from the Centre! So much went on between the lines of those notes during her four years attendance, but even this is as nothing compared with all the real work that went on in the often agonising hours of darkness at home, as she learned to face herself, her fear and to find her power.

## Katherina's Comments to the Medical Profession

Katherina is completely convinced that patients should be informed of their diagnosis, but feels that more effort should be made by the medical profession to help the patient through the ensuing depression. She believes that doctors should never give estimates of life expectancy as this is the equivalent of a death sentence, is profoundly damaging and can become a self-fulfilling prophesy merely because the patient is so undermined and suggestible. One of the ways to partially alleviate the despair of this time is to be positive and to provide lots of information about what the patient can do to help him or herself. Most importantly, though, the doctor must be kind, patient and sympathetic and explain the diagnosis and proposed treatment as many times as it takes for the patient to understand. She also feels that cancer needs to lose its special status as the leprosy of our times and be treated like any other illness.

She wishes and hopes that doctors can come to the point of supporting their patients in the trying of non-invasive therapies before launching into the routine practice of surgery, chemotherapy and radiotherapy: these should be saved for the last resort, as opposed to being the first line of treatment. Even where such therapies have to be used she is sure that prognosis and side effects could be improved by preparing the patient both psychologically and physically. Her most fervent wish however is that doctors would learn when to stop. Katherina suggests that the main problem is the doctor's own fear of the reality of the situation and the fact that they cannot themselves face the thought of death: either their own or the patient's. She believes that patients should have the right to choose to die rather than have treatment, and that doctors must address this area of fear in themselves. This would enable dialogue between doctors and their patients about the possibility of allowing death to occur in a spontaneous and conscious manner; not in a great frenzy of fear and panic, or once the patient has been reduced to a physical and psychological heap.

Her definition of a good doctor or therapist is someone who can explain all the different aspects of your illness and all the different possibilities for treatment, but most importantly of all, who can show you that there is much that you can do if you want to. She deeply acknowledges the superb care of her own GP pinpointing as his greatest attribute the fact that he was "big enough" to go on seeing and supporting her when he had no medical treatment left to offer her. Time and again patients say that that is the very moment when they most need their doctor; more often than not (either because they feel they have failed or have nothing to offer) it's also the very time when the doctor will stop seeing the patient or drastically reduce the frequency of visits.

## Dr Latto's Comments

Dr Latto is a remarkably forward thinking GP. He is completely convinced about the relationship between negative or depressed states of mind and poor physical health. He says that he has often witnessed and even predicted the breakdown of the physical health of his patients following traumatic life events which have caused severe emotional or nervous shock. He quotes the example of a couple whose house was burgled with the loss of all the husband's professional photographic equipment and current work. The husband was devastated by the occurence. Within a few days he had a coronary thrombosis and died. His wife, who had been in a seven year remission from breast cancer then rapidly deteriorated, swiftly developing metastatic disease from which she died within two months of her husband's death.

Dr Latto, in the treatment of his patients, therefore places great emphasis on helping them maintain mental equilibrium, or where possible a really determined and positive frame of mind. He is very keen on the use of any counselling and visualisation techniques which create a better self-image and sense of potency in the patient. Quite separately to this he emphasises the importance of helping the patient to feel good! This may sound like stating the obvious, but is remarkably often ignored by doctors who concentrate on the treating of the objective disease state, and not helping the patient through the subjective reality of their illness. This approach includes getting patients to find out what really makes them feel good, encouraging them to get involved in any practices which create a state of wellbeing (as opposed to feelings of guilt or pressure). He feels that in such a state, emotional problems (especially fear) recede and patients are better able to take the practical difficulties of their situations into their stride. In other words the negative feedback loop of illness/diagnosis/depression/ exacerbation of illness can be broken in this way.

One of the ways Dr Latto is convinced people can make themselves feel better is through eating a lighter diet. He believes that most of us consume vastly in excess of our protein and fat requirements and that all of us could cut back greatly in these areas with an ensuing improvement in state of mind and health. He believes this becomes especially important in cancer patients as tumours are 'protein hungry'; and that, by cutting back to optimum levels of protein for the individual the rate of tumour growth can be curbed. He cites the practice within cancer research laboratories of keeping the experimental animals on very high protein diets in order to maintain their tumours which have been induced by carcinogens. If they are kept on their normal diet the tumours often disappear!

He establishes the correct level of protein for a given individual by keeping a close eye on their weight and energy levels when putting them on such diets. The aim is to create the greatest improvement in energy level and sense of well-being, without causing weight loss beyond the optimum weight for the given individual. Obviously where patients have already lost weight due to their disease, the diet is modified accordingly to allow weight gain to occur. In these cases the patient must be given extra protein but extra calories are mainly given in the form of carbohydrate. Dr Latto is utterly convinced of the causal relationship between the unbalanced, contaminated and predominantly carnivorous diets of the West and high cancer levels, and therefore stresses the importance of healthy diet to all his patients as a preventative measure. He in fact takes a stronger line on diet than Bristol, encouraging cancer patients to stay on a very strict 'clean' diet and not to revert to old habits after three months! He does not prescribe grape diets himself but will support patients through the grape diet if they wish to try it.

Dr Latto also has very positive feelings about the use of Iscador, based both on the research of its use and his own experience with cancer patients, many of whom have experienced improved health following its use. However, he has only limited enthusiasm for vitamin and mineral supplementation, feeling that whilst supplementation may have a place initially, it may be greatly reduced once the diet has been corrected.

In summary then he cannot help but conclude that Katherina's case bears out all his theories and that The Bristol Cancer Help Centre has done Katherina nothing but good. She has had no side effects from any of the treatments or diet, has beaten her disease, and is so strong that each week she inspires, supports and encourages many other people to face and cope with their disease as bravely as she has done, in whatever way is right for each one of them individually. Neither Katherina nor Dr Latto would ever advise against any mainstream treatment, but both would hope that by giving sufficient loving support, encouragement and a sense of positivity that they could create the security in which an individual could make an informed decision about treatment which was really true to their innermost feelings.

## Chapter 5

# Reg Flower
## Medical History

(*Birth Date*: 5 March 1931)

*Supplied by Dr I.C. Murison (GP) and Mr Ron Hiles (Surgeon).*

I have only made a summary of Reg's medical history because of its complexity, and because Reg goes into great detail about his medical experience in the telling of his story.

1976 — Excision of a rodent ulcer from his back.

1981 — Excision of malignant melanoma from his chest.

1981 — 1982 Suffered badly with ankylosing spondylosis (a disease involving the gradual joining up of the bones in the neck with ensuing pain and entrapment of nerves).

1982 — Anterior cervical fusion, and excision of intervertebral discs (C3/4 and C4/5) to relieve arm and neck pain.

1982 — Appearance of secondary melanoma in the lymph glands under his right arm. Excision of these glands and simultaneous repair of vertebra venous fistula (caused by the previous operation).

1983 — Removal of second rodent ulcer from left side of chest.

## Reg's Story

Reg was born and brought up in Pewsey on the Salisbury Plain. He was the oldest of three children. His father was in the army and so he went to the local army school. During his childhood his father was posted to Palestine. The family was to have followed him out there, but war broke out in the meantime. His father didn't return for five years and during this period his parents divorced. He left school at 14 to become apprenticed to an undertaker but was laid off after a year because there was insufficient work! He then got a job in the NAAFI stores for a while and after that became the local cinema projectionist. At 17 he went into the air force and became an electrician. He married at twenty, but a month after his wedding he was posted to Gibraltar to install the wiring for the military early warning systems.

From there he was posted still further afield to the Suez Canal. Here he had to run a power station on the side of the canal which supplied electricity to all the army and air force bases. He also had to maintain the power lines going out across the desert, which was pretty hair-raising because he would often get shot at in the process! He came out of the air force after five years and returned home to his wife. They had three children during the six years after his return but they had spent such a long time apart by that point their relationship was somewhat strained. He feels that this began to change his nature because previously he had been a very relaxed type. He began to feel very tense and pressured and thinks that this is when he began to develop a short temper.

He brought his family up in Bath. His parents both came from Bath originally, and so Reg had relatives there. He got a job with Lucas' car electrics department immediately after leaving the air force, but unfortunately this job didn't last long and work became so hard to find that he had to take a job in in Chippenham, again in car electrics. This involved him setting out at 5am and getting home at 10pm every day because he had to rely on public transport. He did this seven days a week for five years! He eventually got a better paid job, though still in Chippenham. This was as a factory maintenance electrician. He stayed there for another five years still working seven days a week, but at least managed to save up enough to buy a motor bike at this stage and so the travelling was a little less problematical. It was while he was there that he saw an advert for a job in Bath as a fruit machine mechanic. This job not only involved no travel, but paid the same wages for five days that he had been earning in seven. He just could not believe this opportunity had come his way, so he jumped at it. He was to stay in that job for over twenty years.

Now that Reg spent more time at home, the cracks in the marriage became a lot more evident. What aggravated the situation still further was that his work took him into clubs and bars, giving much more fertile territory for his wife's anxiety. The final straw was in 1968 when the firm asked Reg to spend his weekdays in Hampshire so that he could oversee the setting up of a new factory. At this point his wife's fears became a self-fulfilling prophecy. He did have an affair which led to their divorce in 1971 and to Reg's second marriage to his present wife Cath.

Cath already had four children. Reg was very happy in his new marriage, but life became very stressful in those early days because of coordinating the movements of seven children between their respective parents, sometimes amidst not the friendliest of atmospheres. The children also got quite skilful at 'winding up' the various parents and setting one against the other. They also had to contend with punk and skinhead phases which frightened the lives out of them! Still there were plenty of good times like when all nine of them went for a caravan holiday in Wales with two cars, tents and the most enormous caravan. Mercifully the children all got on very well and so their teenage years were really very happy. The youngest is now in her early twenties and married and all the others live independently too, so Cath and Reg have really had much more time together over the last few years.

In 1980 things started going very sour for Reg. He became the victim of extremely severe stress at work with devastating consequences. All his life he had had a tendency to grow moles. They would start as red blisters and then either disappear or turn black. In the Autumn of 1980 he noticed that one of his moles on his breastbone just kept on growing. It started off about the size of the end of his finger and got bigger and bigger over the course of a year until it was the size of an old fashioned half crown. It looked odd to Reg because it was such an intense, blue black colour and looked almost as if it was wet under the skin. He ignored it for some time as he was preoccupied with his work situation. Eventually, after a lot of pestering from Cath, he decided he'd better go and see his doctor. The doctor didn't like the look of it at all and sent him to see a skin specialist immediately. This was possible for Reg because he was covered by medical insurance. The consultant dermato-logist took a biopsy then and there under local anaesthetic. Within two days he was telephoned with the news that he had a malignant melanoma and that he must come back into hospital immediately to see a surgeon. That turned out to be Mr Ron Hiles who saw him and reassured him that there was nothing to worry about, he would just need to remove a small bit of skin around the melanoma.

In August 1981 he came into a nursing home in Clifton, Bristol. He went down to the theatre at about midday but came round from his anaesthetic late at night. The first thing he became aware of was the church bell in Clifton striking twelve midnight. Its gloomy note made him feel frightened and very lonely. The second thing he noticed was an enormous pad on his chest. He remembers thinking, "That's funny, what's all that doing there" and then he dropped off to sleep again. The next realisation in the morning was that his leg was "playing up something cruel". Mr Hiles had had to take such a large piece of skin from Reg's chest that a skin graft had become necessary and so he had taken the graft from Reg's thigh. Unfortunately, because there was so little flesh under the area which had been excised over the breast bone the graft didn't take and the skin was rejected. So Reg's stay in hospital became very drawn out as the area slowly healed naturally, forming a new layer of scar tissue. This meant that Mr Hiles had to come and clean and trim the wound every day which was extremely painful and nauseating. Reg is sure that he intuitively learnt self-hypnosis at this stage in order to get himself through these ordeals. He would pick a spot on the ceiling and concentrate on it to the exclusion of all else until the dressing was done, thereby significantly reducing his awareness of the whole situation.

The skin on his leg took a very long time to heal too and is still very thin and easily damaged. On the surface Reg took the diagnosis quite calmly. He says, "I'm not the sort of person to be horrified or shocked. Surprised yes, but it didn't really throw me particularly". At the time this happened he considered himself in A1 shape physically so it was very odd to be a patient, suddenly requiring all this attention. He does say though that a part of him knew that it was cancer from the time the patch began to grow and he thinks that is the real reason he put off going to the doctors for such a long time.

He hadn't really consciously appreciated what a bad effect the work situation was having on him. At that stage he had worked with the fruit machine company for eighteen years (since 1962). He had worked himself up from the very bottom over the years.

By this stage he was in charge of a work force of fifty and the design and manufacturing for the whole firm. At one point, a few years earlier when it looked as if the whole factory would have to close and everybody lose their jobs, he had had the idea that he could make at least part of the production into cottage industry. He did this by changing the designs so that individual components could be made by the workers at their homes, thereby obviating the need to keep up such large premises and so much machinery. He then co-ordinated the smooth running of the operation and made sure it was a success. He didn't feel that the firm ever really gave him credit for this salvage operation, but he was satisfied in the knowledge that he was to get his reward in 1980 in the form of a directorship. This had been promised to him by the chairman. Reg felt this promotion was absolutely in order and was looking forward to a bit of financial freedom too.

Reg describes his old self as quite a fiery type. He was easily annoyed and would 'blow his top' if provoked, but as far as he was concerned that was it, as soon as it was out it was over. He will admit that in the years leading up to 1980 he had a few heated discussions with the directors about the feasibility of some of their proposals, but nothing that he would have called a major rift occured. He was amazed then, not long before his promotion was due, to be called up in front of the directors and told in no uncertain terms that they were very displeased with him and his general attitude. They even wanted him to sign a form which amounted to his 'first public warning'. Apparently this involves agreeing to the charges which have been levelled and if one gets three of these, dismissal becomes inevitable. Reg was incredibly hurt and very angry. As far as he was concerned he'd sweat blood for that firm. Whenever anybody was off sick he would stand in in their place in order to keep production deadlines. There wasn't one job in the factory he couldn't do. He would even stay on in the evenings long after everyone else had gone home to get the work done and arrive there again at 7 o'clock in the morning to sort things out before the others arrived.

In fact he realises that he probably had a tendency in all areas of life to take on too much responsibility and was in general a very poor delegator. He also realises that he was really a work-aholic and that his behaviour had quite a 'driven' quality to it.

He genuinely believed that no one else could or would do it if he didn't and so it always seemed absolutely necessary to 'get on and do'. None the less he had felt completely in the right during the various 'run-ins' he had had with the management because he knew the set up infinitely better in practical terms than they did. To be given a 'black mark' in this way hit him extremely hard — with uncannily literal sequelae!

He didn't sign the paper and over the next few months it became a battle of nerves. At any excuse the management took away more and more of his responsibility until he was literally sitting around with nothing to do. They effectively froze him out and in the worst way possible, because for a doer like Reg to be twiddling his thumbs was absolute murder, not to mention the agony of seeing all his carefully set up plans and schemes being messed up in one way or another by those who had taken his place. He didn't really take this upset anywhere as he didn't want to burden Cath who was already looking after their combined brood and neither did he have the sort of friends he could open up to in that way. It never occured to him to go to his doctor nor that it might contribute to his becoming so seriously ill.

Reg now thinks that, if he'd been a bit more canny and less full of righteous indignation, things needn't have got as bad as they did but he just couldn't bear to back down when he knew he was in the right and was being treated so appallingly. It sounds very much, reading between the lines, as if Reg must have been a terrible threat to the other managers because of his extraordinary application. He says that he was the kind of person who would take somebody saying that a job couldn't be done as a challenge — and he'd always prove them wrong. The other big blow was that the chairman, who had promised Reg the directorship in the first place, was by this time an old and close personal friend of Reg's, but kept a very low profile during the whole affair. Reg felt that he could have changed things but he didn't.

His operation and all the ensuing problems kept him off work for three months and even then, he now realises, he went back to work too soon. He returned in the Christmas of 1981 only to find that his next problem was that he was getting tingling and numbness all down his arms. Mr Hiles, who was keeping a close eye on him, was absolutely sure that this was nothing to do with the cancer so he went to see an orthopaedic surgeon who said that it was caused by trapping of the nerves in his neck and could be cured by an operation on his neck to join two of the vertebrae together. Because the arm problem was slowing him down so much he thought he'd better go ahead and get this done. It didn't sound like too big a deal anyway. He'd had spinal surgery as a younger man for disc problems in the lumbar lower back region and had got over that just fine.

So in the May of 1982 he went in to hospital. To his absolute horror he woke up in intensive care after the operation to discover that the surgeon had operated from the front and not the back of his neck as he had imagined he would, and that he had effectively cut his throat! What was also horrific was that that first night in intensive care he came round to see two nurses chatting to each other about their boyfriends over his bed. He desperately wanted some human contact at that moment but couldn't really talk. He tried to smile but when they saw he was awake they said, "Oh look, he's coming round — better give him an injection". Whereupon he suddenly had the bed clothes whipped back and a hypodermic needle stuck in his leg. The injection itself was extremely painful for Reg, but even worse was the feeling of complete dehumanisation, not to mention terror and loneliness. He wishes to make a heart felt plea to nurses everywhere, to remember that, even if the patient may appear drowsy or not quite 'with it', their mind, hearing and feelings may well be totally intact.

As with his other operation he also had a double wound, because they had taken the bone chips to join the two vertebrae from his iliac crest (hip region) and so again he had two lots of discomfort to cope with. The final straw when he eventually got up off his back, was to discover that during the operation nerves in his neck had been cut which affected his lips, tongue and eye on the right side of his face. This meant that his eye drooped and he couldn't talk or eat properly. Yet another blow to come was that during his convalescent phase he noticed that every time he got worked up or excited there was a squeaking noise coming from his neck. He soon realised that this was related to his heart rate. It transpired that damage done to an artery and vein in the neck had left a little passageway between the two vessels and that blood was oscillating to and fro between them. With a low heart beat this wasn't noticeable, but as the rate and pressure went up he could hear this funny noise.

The facial problems have improved with time and I certainly didn't notice any asymmetry to his face but there are still words that he can't pronounce properly. He says with tears glistening in his eyes that he would never ever go through that again. If he had had the slightest inkling of what it really entailed, he would have put up with the original problem. He was obviously deeply traumatised by the whole incident. He actually turned the 'squeak' problem to his advantage before it was treated because he used to use it, bio-feedback style, to learn how to bring down his heart rate and blood pressure once he started learning stress reduction techniques. Thank God the operation did cause some slight improvement of his arm problem but sadly this time he didn't get back to work.

In the July of that year, when he was just about over the worst of this trauma, he went along to Mr Hiles for his routine check up. Mr Hiles discovered a big lump under his right arm which he said would have to be operated upon immediately because it was a secondary. When he mentioned the squeak to Mr Hiles, a vascular surgeon was called in, and he too decided that further surgery was inevitable. So to Reg's horror, in the August of 1982, it was back to the operating theatre once again; this time for a six hour operation with two surgeons working simultaneously on the two different problems. Reg thinks that it was the stress of the first neck operation which triggered his secondary melanoma.

Almost predictably there were further complications after this operation too. Because Reg had to have all the lymph nodes cleared from under his arm, this meant disrupting the flow of lymph from his arm into his body. Normally after this operation, the lymph finds new pathways after ten or so days allowing the drain to be removed. But for poor old Reg the area just kept on draining and draining for weeks at the rate of about a pint a day! To add to the complications the tube on the drain kept on blocking, causing his shoulder to swell enormously and so Reg had to keep on going in to hospital to have a new drain put in. Eventually he got so sick of this that he decided to do it himself! He would pull it out, blow it through, then microwave it to sterilise it and stick it back into his arm!!! The medical mind boggles. It is amazing he didn't die of septicaemia! In fact 'do-it-yourself Reg' even made a little sling for his drain so that he could wear it under his shirt and went on a camping holiday in France for three weeks with the drain in-situ.

Two days before the end of the holiday the drainage finally began to slow down and on the last day he decided to disconnect the whole thing and go scuba diving. Once again the fact that he didn't get seriously infected is a miracle. However he says that after two hours of diving for sea urchins he was so exhausted that he collapsed, unable to walk when he got out of the sea. He had to lie on the sand like a beached whale for an hour or so to get his strength back. He got away with it and didn't need to continue with the drainage, but for many months his hand remained extremely swollen and often quite rigid, making it difficult to bend his fingers. His other problem was that the operation to remove the bone chips from his hip had left his leg numb and at one point on holiday he'd fallen over and taken a large patch of skin off his leg without even realising it. Because of his run down state it took a very long time to heal.

When he got home in the late autumn he felt thoroughly demoralised and depressed. He had dropped from 15 to 10 stone (210 — 140 lbs) and felt as weak as a kitten. He knew only too well that the arrival of his secondaries meant that his chances of long-term survival were drastically reduced and he looked like a terminally ill patient. Getting through the winter of 1982 was a terrible struggle. The first glimmer of hope came shortly after Christmas of that year when he came across an article on holistic medicine in his newspaper. His interest was aroused instantly. He wrote to the paper the same day and got a reply with the address of ANAC (The Association for New Approaches to Cancer). ANAC put him in touch with the Cancer Help Centre as he lived so close by. On January 4th 1983 he walked into the old centre at Downfield Road and tells me, brimming over with emotion, that on walking through the door he immediately felt as if he had been lifted a foot off the floor. That poor sweet man had been through this whole ordeal without sharing his feelings with a soul. He says he has never looked back from that day on. He can hardly describe the feeling he had. He says he felt freed, like a man being let out of prison. He felt so at ease with everyone and so relaxed and safe for the first time in months because the place was so crowded with people in the same state as him.

He recalls that the house was so full that once the food had been prepared in the kitchen, they would have to move tables and chairs into the kitchen to seat everybody for lunch and even then there were people sitting on the stairs. There was the most wonderfully intense feeling of support and solidarity that was almost palpable. Without even speaking everyone there was completely united in their fight against their common enemies of fear, loneliness and disease. He made up his mind then and there that whatever else happened he would never again have another operation. He says that the feeling was more than just relief, it was as if some part of his being which had never been nourished or recognised before, was suddenly completely at home.

He got straight into the diet and kept on it absolutely strictly for six months. He also had very intensive counselling initially, going to see Ludi How twice weekly at her own home. He had a tremendous amount of material to 'work through' because of all the difficult unexpressed feelings which had accumulated over the years. Through this process he came to accept completely the role he had played in the creating of his own problems at work. He realised that he just couldn't go on blaming other people indefinitely for everthing which was happening to him. At some point he had to accept at least part of the responsibility. He learnt that if he never told anybody what was going on inside it was no wonder people kept trampling all over his finer feelings. Also, vitally for Reg, he finally learnt to have some trust in other people and began to delegate. He had to give up the belief that he was the only person who could do things in his world.

The counselling did more than make him just realise these things, he actually changed his way of being drastically; so much so, in fact, that people who knew him before can't believe that it's the same person because he is now so much more sensitive, emotional and open to his and other peoples feelings. His priority has shifted entirely from 'doing' to 'being' and his goal has changed from achieving to looking after the quality of his time. He likes the 'new him' much better. He also finds that his relationships with Cath and the children have really deepened as a result of these changes.

He got on really well with imaging, but found relaxation and meditation nigh on impossible at first, unless he was physically exhausted. He thinks that the visualisation came so easily to him because as a designer one is visualising all the time anyway. He used to use the image of a golden healing globe which he would take all over his body cleaning up any debris or cancer. When he had taken it everywhere he would take it to his liver and empty out the contents there to be 'incinerated'. He says no-one ever told him this, he just had the feeling that the liver was the place to dump it all. A time came when he just could not conjure up this image any more. Instead the only image that would come was that of a bearded shepherd in a brown sacking robe who was gently herding his flock of sheep. One thing was constant, which was that the shepherd was always smiling. This character became a very comforting guide and friend for Reg even though he never spoke but most significant of all, his arrival became symbolic for Reg of the end of his illness.

Initially Reg was extremely sceptical about healing, thinking it was 'a load of old rubbish'. However he was actually very surprised at how much he got out of it. There was a healer there called Irene Stevens the day he visited the Centre. He reluctantly went in to see her. She told him to shut his eyes and relax. The first thing he felt was terrific heat from her hands and then the most uncanny and powerful vibration all through himself. He opened his eyes in amazement only to discover that she didn't even have her hands on him! After she had finished he felt wonderfully exhilarated and this continued to happen every time she gave him healing. He says that he carried on seeing her at her home too, and when he came out of the house he would be singing at the top of his voice — this was extraordinary for him because up till then he'd never sung a note in his life! Again, as with nearly all these people, he says that he has tried other healers who have done absolutely nothing for him at all. He says if he hadn't had that amazing experience the first time he probably wouldn't have bothered again as it would have confirmed his expectations. So he would really urge people to keep looking until they get the right healer for them.

Later on he joined a healing group in his area. This consisted of about seven people and was led by an ex-barrister who had given up his practice to work exclusively in the healing field. He would first lead the group in meditation and guided imagery. Then they would form a healing circle once they were all in a very relaxed and receptive state. The group would also send absent healing to others they knew who were in deep trouble of any sort. Reg stayed with the group all through 1985 and in fact used this resource to help his son in law who had developed a cancer of his lymph glands. To Reg's amazement the ex-barrister told Reg that he was a healer himself. This was very funny for Reg considering his initial scepticism. He did however help prove it to himself later because he is sure he saved his cat's life once after he became poisoned accidentally. After many days of intensive care from the vet all hope had really been lost. Reg would not accept this and sat for many hours giving the cat healing. This put the cat into a very long sleep, after which he was able to eat again and slowly came back to his normal self.

Interestingly the same cat seems to be a bit of a healer itself because the matron from a hospital very close to Reg's house says that the cat comes in most days and always seems to make a bee-line for the sickest person. He then jumps on their laps, snuggles in and sits there purring and licking them! She says that many a patient has been extremely cheered by this gentle presence.

He worked out many other ways to tackle his practical problems too. He had realised that if he squeezed his hand he could dissipate some of the fluid in his hand and arm, so he took this one stage further and used to carry a tennis ball round with him that he would keep squeezing as he felt the pressure building up. He had to change the tennis ball every three days though because he would burst them after this long! This got expensive so he eventually he got himself a solid foam ball. His next thought was that it was probably the increase in circulation that the squeezing caused which helped get rid of the fluid so maybe if he generally speeded up his circulation the problem would subside still further. He thought he could achieve this by running. At this point he was still very sick and weak. He says that at the first attempt he collapsed at his garden gate but after a few weeks he was managing two miles in thirteen minutes! He would do this at five am, be back at the house by five-fifteen and then relax and meditate until six o'clock. The focus for his meditation was to concentrate on his breathing, imagining that he was breathing out through the palms of his hands. He says this was such a hard thing to imagine that it kept his mind beautifully occupied. After he had completed this routine he would then shower and have his breakfast. Eventually he bought his own exercise bicycle and uses this for combined exercise and imaging time. He says he can travel down country lanes on it smelling the flowers and hearing the birds, or even float on clouds across Salisbury Plain if he wants to — all from his garden shed in Bath!

Reg used the biofeedback meter to help him learn to find a truly relaxed state initially. He got quite good at it at the Centre and decided to put himself to the test at home. Try as he might he couldn't even get a reading on it at home because there were so many stress-inducing stimuli around him that he just couldn't let go. Of course, being Reg, he couldn't let the challenge go either and he persevered and persevered until he managed it. Now he can just get into a chair and go into a deep relaxation with ease which he would never have believed possible before. The meter works by giving a higher reading the less tense an individual is. He says that with new-comers who are very tense and embarrassed by their inability to get the needle to move at all a good trick is to come up to them and give their hand a reassuring squeeze. Nine times out of ten this momentary relaxation sends the needle zooming up. This immediately demonstrates to them the state of mind which is being sought and that it really is possible for them to achieve it.

Reg now, like so many of the people who have benefitted from the approach, gives time every week to help others who are just starting on this path. His contribution is to go to the Centre on Sunday evening to welcome in the new resident patients. They say every time that to meet one other patient who has recovered is worth twenty doctors and counsellors talking about theoretical possibilities! He finds over and over again that the first reaction of the new patients is the liberation they feel in even being able to mention the word cancer. Once given permission to talk, their distress comes flooding out and he is often there late into the night listening as the patients and their relatives unburden themselves.

In these ways Reg gradually returned to health and actually got himself back to work in the spring of 1983. Even the people at the Centre were amazed at his recovery, and someone confided in him later that nobody really thought that he would make it as he had looked so ghastly when he'd first arrived. He started a few hours at a time and gradually worked his way up to full time again. However, there were two more big knocks to come for Reg. In the May of that year Cath was diagnosed as having a malignant melanoma too. Since Reg's operation Cath and Reg had kept a very close eye on each other's skin. Cath had complained of some itching on her back and lo and behold there was a mole about the size of the end of a pencil. When Reg heard the diagnosis he wept. He was even more upset when he saw her back after the operation because she too had to have an enormous excision of skin and underlying tissue. At least this time he was able to let his feelings out, and they had all the benefits of his experience to get them through. However the Centre itself wasn't for Cath. Reg thinks he took her there at the wrong time. The minute she got out of hospital he rushed her straight over there. It just depressed her still further and she actually ran out of the place crying. She says, "All I could see were people that were dying". The long and short of it is that she hadn't made her own decision to go and so Reg's approach and timing had been wrong. Happily, Cath has remained very well, and at the time I saw her was in very good health and spirits.

As if Reg didn't have enough on his plate there was yet another blow to come from work. He was called in and told that the firm would have to cut his wages by half. This was nothing to do with his illness and was justified on the basis that the firm was once again in deep financial trouble. Reg went away and being his usual resourceful self immediately came up with a plan whereby they could save four times as much as they would by cutting his wages. What they were intending to pay him was less than the mechanics! They weren't at all interested in his proposition and he just decided at this stage that he had lost all interest in working for them. So he decided to go for redundancy instead: he's sure this was what they were after anyway. He got the bare minimum redundancy money of £1000 after twenty years' service.

At the time this was very hard to swallow, despite his new found strength. After all, this was only five months into his self-help programme. He says that if he hadn't had the Centre at that point he knows that would have been the end of him. When it happened he just fell back into their arms while he licked his wounds. He didn't even try to 'cope'. Now, however, he thinks it is the best thing that ever happened because he has got himself into a highly lucrative business which he runs from home. He also helps other people to make money in their spare time calling himself a 'secondary income specialist'.

He somehow also has enough time to do ambulance driving. He picks old people up in the morning to take them into a psychiatric day centre and then takes them home again at tea time. This is rather a different Reg from the ambitious managing director! He says that he surreptitiously gives them healing as he lifts them in and out of the ambulance now and he often notices how this quietens the agitated patients. Not surprisingly they all adore him and it seems to be the best bit of the day for them! He knows that he will carry on doing this even if he does become financially independent, because he gets such a boost out of seeing the lift that he gives the patients. He cannot verbalise or analyse at all what he thinks healing is, but says that it is just an extremely loving feeling that comes over him. He's actually rather embarrassed about doing it or talking about it and would never set himself up as a healer, preferring to give it without advertising the fact.

Rather like Joan, Reg never really contemplated the possibility of death. He says that he was too caught up in feeling sorry for himself and finding practical solutions to the various problems that each new operation brought about. He has never felt the need to interpret any of the new feelings he felt at the Centre in religious terms. The only contact he has had with the Church is that during his recuperation period he used to often feel drawn to going to sit in the peace of Bath Abbey.

If anything could have been different for Reg he wishes that he could have been better prepared psychologically for the medical procedures he underwent. Not only would this have avoided the nightmare situation in the intensive care unit, but it would also have given him a chance to give informed consent to having the operations in the first place! He is very glad that nobody ever gave him any sort of prognosis or full blown detail about the seriousness of his condition. He has never really asked Mr Hiles for his opinion of the Centre or discussed his beliefs about its benefits but has heard through the grapevine to his great satisfaction that Mr Hiles has since referred several patients there himself. His summary of what is special about the Centre is that it is the love and patience of all involved there; the fact that everyone on the staff gives minute attention to every individual need, fear and query. He does feel that theoretically this is transferable into the N.H.S. context, but feels it is impossible within the present climate because of the lack of time available to the doctors and nurses to spend with individual patients. He even fears that the Centre may fall into the same trap if in their desire to reach more people they have too many people there at once.

What Reg feels he has gained is health, peace of mind and a completely new character. He feels he now considers others in a way that he never did before. He has a new kind of confidence which he never had before and is eternally grateful to Pat and Penny for their courage in setting up the Centre.

## Mr Hiles' Comments

It is impossible for Mr Hiles to say whether there is anything unusual about Reg's recovery, because melanoma is such an unpredictable disease. He says he has had several patients in the thousand or so cases of melanoma he has seen who have done remarkably well for no obvious reason.

He has been very tempted at times to believe that there is a connection between life events and the development of melanoma, and has expected research to prove a connection between our mental state, the health of our defence systems and the incidence of and recovery from melanoma. However, recently a very distinguished scientific friend who has spent his whole life looking for the defence mechanisms involved in keeping melanoma cells in check, has told him that he has had to come to the conclusion that there just aren't any. The more sceptical part of him suggests that we have a tendency to say that illnesses are caused by stress until we know the real cause. Whatever the aetiology, what is most alarming is that the incidence of melanoma is increasing by ten per cent annually and the most popular explanation for this is the increased exposure of the British to intense sunlight and sun lamps. It is certainly interesting to note that Reg and Cath used to own a sun ray lamp, and would spend all the time they could roasting themselves in the Mediterranean. They threw out the lamp after Cath, too, developed her melanoma. While there is no absolute evidence about the danger of these lamps Mr Hiles intuitively distrusts them. He says, "Ultra-violet is incredibly strong stuff. It causes polythene to denature twice as fast as normal and will also completely discharge static electricity."

Mr Hiles feels that the alternative cancer world is 'groping in the dark', but that so too, is orthodox medicine. He recalls that the GP who delivered his children told him many years ago, that after fifty years of practice, he could predict which of his patients would get cancer. Initially Mr Hiles thought this rather clever and probably very wise, but as he has accumulated experience of his own, he feels rather less inclined to subscribe to the 'cancer personality' theory. Of course, he says, there is so much else to take into consideration as life gets more and more sophisticated, complex and dominated by scientific technology that maybe the days are past when personality type alone can be used as a predictor.

He feels that cancer is an extremely complex multi-factorial disease and that there are likely to be hundreds of different diseases, depending on the inter-reaction between a specific cancer, and a specific host in a specific environment. He even describes one case where he was aware of three different sub-species of cancerous cells growing with entirely different characteristics in the same person. Another vital point that Mr Hiles makes is that in most types of cancer we do not even know the natural history of the disease — in other words, what would happen if we gave no treatment at all? He has a distinct feeling that it is quite probable that it will eventually be proved that the medical treatment of cancer probably affects prognosis very little — if at all. This certainly seems to be the case with breast cancer. In the whole history of the surgical, pharmacological and radiotherapeutic treatment of breast cancer there has been no overall improvement in survival rates. This again highlights the very primitive state of our understanding of cancer!

As far as the giving of prognosis is concerned, Mr Hiles says that he will, if pressed, give individuals statistics for their chances of survival, but always points out to them that this is pretty meaningless as he has no way of knowing which half of the statistical group an individual will fall into. He would never give an individual their prognosis in terms of years. He says, "I think that's playing God". If people ask him how long they've got he will always say that he has absolutely no idea. At the time of Reg's diagnosis in 1981, based on the thickness of his original tumour, his chance of surviving five years was eighty per cent. However from the point of getting his lymph nodes in 1982 the statistics changed to a fifty per cent chance of his surviving five years. Reg is therefore in the lucky half of the prognostic group, as he has now safely survived the five year period since the appearance of his secondaries with no signs of recurrence. Although he cannot say so categorically, Mr Hiles would certainly like to believe that it is Reg's own efforts and attitude which have enabled him to make such a good recovery, and he would certainly not try to dissuade Reg from believing this.

Mr Hiles is very much in favour of the supportive elements of alternative treatment of cancer. He tries himself to be very supportive in terms of his own attitude to the disease. He is extremely careful "never to take anybody's props away". He will point out to patients, that while they have a disease that they know about, he may just as easily be suffering from something he doesn't know about, like ischaemic heart disease. This means he could fall down dead tomorrow making his own prognosis worse than theirs. He therefore constantly plays on the fact that none of us can know when or how our 'time will come' and that we must all therefore live for one day at a time, (which is what he tries to do). He does not particularly direct his patients to alternative treatment, but will never actively advise against it. What he does feel is essential, however, is close communication between all doctors and therapists involved in the management of a case. This is because he feels that great efforts should be made to ensure that patients are never given conflicting advice. In other words, he feels that the doctors and practitioners should battle out the pros and cons of the giving of different sorts of advice between themselves and present a united front, rather than expecting the poor patient to sort these out with possible ensuing demoralisation, feelings of betrayal of one side or the other or, worse still, alienation from both camps.

On the subject of whether mental attitude has any part in the outcome of physical disease, Mr Hiles says, "I work on the premise that it does — I certainly feel in my bones that the attitude you might be able to impart to a patient has a part to play in their recovery". He would be very interested to see the results of trials done to show the different medical outcomes of patients receiving exactly the same orthodox treatments, but from different doctors and hospitals. He is quite sure that these would show that response to treatment varies widely from doctor to doctor. However, he thinks that you can go too far in trying to influence patients' attitudes. One of his criticisms of the Centre is that he thinks that individuals' hopes are sometimes raised too high. He actually thinks that the degree of positivism an individual musters is in fact in direct proportion to the degree of negativity they feel. This is certainly in line with my observation, that almost all the patients who do really well at the Centre are those who genuinely appreciate the danger they are in, experience their terror or outrage and as a result make concrete resolutions to beat their disease.

He is quite clear that faith healing or spiritual healing really does happen although he thinks probably not nearly as often as is claimed. He doesn't understand it at all but is completely open to it. He would never actually refer someone to a healer however, feeling this would have to come from them. He is well aware of the benefits of meditation and relaxation as he practises these himself in the context of his Christian faith. As such, therefore, he has never thought of meditation as a technique and finds this view of it rather strange and mechanistic. He cannot imagine meditation outside the context of faith.

He thinks that vitamin and mineral supplementation is unnecessary if one eats a healthy diet, and would generally recommend an unprocessed healthy diet to all his patients.

In general then, it appeared to me that Mr Hiles was extremely open to all possibilities for both the treatment and aetiology of cancer. He firmly believes in the importance of positive mental attitude in the recovery process and takes great care to make his patients feel as supported as possible.

## Dr Murison's comments

Dr Murison clearly remembers a consultation in 1979 when Reg told him that he felt as if he was 'going to burst'. He recalls that Reg was struggling with issues raised by his divorce, especially in relation to its divisive effect on his children. When secondaries appeared within a year of the diagnosis in 1981, he felt, "Very gloomy about such a notoriously nasty tumour in a man of his age". He knew little about the Cancer Help Centre when Reg told him he wanted to attend in early 1983 but raised no objection. He was impressed from the start at the very positive attitude to his condition that attendance produced in Reg. However, he was somewhat daunted by the list of vitamins he was asked to prescribe. He aquiesced none the less, despite the fact that Reg came back 'orange as a guinea' a few weeks later from the Beta-carotene he had been given. He states, "His condition regarding his melanoma has varied not at all from the path of recovery since this time, and I expect this to continue". He now has three patients who have attended the Centre with considerable benefit, but cannot say exactly what it is about the approach which works. He suspects that it is not "the ritual of the vitamins", but rather the altered attitude, fear being replaced by confidence and the learning of realistic coping.

He says that, "A sort of calm comes off these patients which is quite noticeable. Cancer patients who know their diagnosis so often generate a feeling of distress in me, so I think this must be how they feel. But Reg Flower and the other two patients cause an altogether different response when they consult." One of his women patients also changed noticeably in her demeanour and use of his service after attending the Centre. Having been extremely fearful and demanding, she ceased to keep asking for home visits, gradually weaned herself off him and then took herself off on a trip to Australia, having decided to live life to the full instead of sitting round feeling dreadful!

He feels that what is communicated between doctor and patients in this subtle way is vital. Confidence, he says, is not just transmitted in words, but also by emotional contact. He feels that if this emotional contact is absent no amount of words will help the patient. He has long believed that ulcers, malignancy, arthritis, thyrotoxicosis, and other illnesses follow a period of crisis, distress or difficult life events. He believes that there is a lot of statistical evidence that this common observation is true. He is distressed by the practice of hospital doctors of informing patients they have cancer without giving them any counselling or 'back up' service. Patients often come back to him devastated, and he is left to repair the damaged morale and cope with the utter hopelessness of the patient and their entire family. Obviously this is particularly bad when the diagnosis of terminal illness has been made, when patients are informed about their impending death without any sort of solace whatsoever.

Dr Murison is in no doubt whatsoever that patients' attitudes to their illnesses is enormously important. For example he compares the recovery time of someone who breaks his leg skiing to someone who has his leg broken as a result of another's carelessness in a car crash, who is therefore both injured and aggrieved. "Guess who gets better first", he says. In his experience it is always the former type of patient who heals quickly with no complications. He feels that this sort of principle applies in all conditions and not least in malignancy. He adds, "Perhaps for the first time I have now seen patients who are confident they can hold the 'Big C' at bay — and perhaps even win!"

In summary he says that, "I have always felt that healing entailed more than 'just giving the right treatment': that a patient's attitude to their condition is almost the most important factor in judging how they will recover. Therefore to be able to change the attitude from negative to positive is really to enable healing instead of just giving treatment."

## Chapter 6

# June Rogers
## Medical History.
(*Birth Date*: 10 June 1932)

The first symptom which June noticed in February 1985 was that she was passing blood in her urine. Her only other symptoms were weight loss and excessive tiredness. June went with these complaints to her GP in Neath, Dr Harris, who then referred her to the general surgeons for their opinion.

Her initial investigation included testing for the presence of a urinary infection which was negative and an intra-venous pyelogram (kidney and bladder x-ray) which also failed to reveal any abnormality. The surgeon, Mr Char, then proceeded to cystoscopy (direct visualisation of the bladder) on the 8th of March 1985, finding an egg sized tumour in the bladder, which he biopsied. Diagnosis was then made of squamous cell carcinoma of the bladder.

Next she was referred to Mr Vaughton, a consultant urologist. He admitted her to his ward on April 3rd so that he could perform a repeat cystoscopy. He too saw a 'necrotic ulcer' in the dome of the bladder and removed what material he could via the cystoscope. The pathology department again confirmed this to be a squamous cell carcinoma with infiltrative cells.

Relevant to this diagnosis is the fact that in 1975 June underwent a total hysterectomy at which time she was noted to have a cyst on her right ovary. It was diagnosed an adeno-carcinoma. This was removed and she was advised thereafter to have a course of radiotherapy to decrease the chances of any spread of the disease. The obvious question in 1985 was whether this bladder tumour was a secondary of her ovarian cancer or a new and distinct primary. Mr Vaughton and the pathologist who made the original diagnosis of the ovarian tumour could come to no definite conclusion about this, but

June herself is quite convinced that it was a new primary, caused by the radiotherapy she had received for the first tumour. June was then discharged with a date to come back to clinic to arrange her treatment.

By the time Mr Vaughton saw June she had already started to attend the Cancer Help Centre. He felt that the tumour was sufficiently well localised that he could offer her an operation to remove it. However, this would also involve removing part of the bladder, which would have caused inconvenience to June for the rest of her life. She refused his offer telling him that she was completely confident that she would heal herself. Mr Vaughton's initial attitude was that she was making a terrible mistake because he was convinced that the tumour would progress rapidly to the inoperable stage. However, in accordance with her wishes he did not pursue the matter, but agreed with her to maintain a regular endoscopic assessment of the tumour, thus keeping the situation under review.

She had her next cystoscopy on June 6th during which further material was removed from the ulcer for pathological investigation. The results of this biopsy were already quite different, showing, "Necrotic calcified material. Acute inflammatory reaction. Few cells are present which may be viable tumour cells." Further cystoscopies performed on September 12th 1985, January 21st 1986 and July 10th 1986 showed the area to be healing and at the last cystoscopy all that remained was a well healed scar with no evidence of underlying tumour. He did not even perform a biopsy at these last three operations as the healing appeared so complete.

## Mr Vaughton's Comments

Mr Vaughton says that he was very surprised by this improving appearance and wonders how much this has been due to his removal of what necrotic material he could on the first two cystoscopies or to June's own efforts. However he would be the first to admit that any partial resection performed via a cystoscope would not constitute a complete medical treatment of this condition. I asked him about his views on the Cancer Help Centre and he replied that he knew very little about it, but feels that any organisation which can provide support, either physical or psychological, to patients with advanced malignant disease seems to have a very useful place in their management. He feels that there is little doubt now that patients with a good and positive mental attitude to their disease will tend to fare better than patients with a negative and defeatist attitude. However he does not feel able to support the use of vitamin and mineral therapy in the treatment of cancer as he is unaware of any satisfactory controlled trials proving their efficacy.

In answer to the question of whether he believes June's own self-healing efforts to have caused her healing he replied that this is almost impossible to assess but does admit that he is rather surprised and very pleased at the way the disease has come under control.

## Comments of Dr Harris — June's GP

Dr Harris does not remember discussing June's prognosis with her, but says that at the time of presentation he would not have been hopeful about a good outcome. He now feels that her prognosis is excellent. He had no fears whatsoever about her attendance at the Centre because of the strict monitoring undertaken by her consultant. He is definitely in favour of self-help, and is supportive of the use of alternative medical treatment as an adjunct to normal medical treatment. He thinks it quite clear that in June's case, her own self-healing efforts have made a difference to the course of her disease. While he was already convinced of the role of self-help in the management of illness he says that June's case has reinforced his inclinations towards alternative methods.

## June's Story

June and her family live in Neath, South Wales. June is Welsh "through and through" and has a wonderful south Walian accent. She has three grown up children, one of whom, her daughter, is a radiographer at Neath hospital. At the time that her illness developed June was running an upholstery business from a shop which formed part of the house she had moved into in 1984. Previously, June had been interested in upholstery as a hobby and did a short apprenticeship with an upholstery firm. After moving into a house with shop premises she decided to establish herself in a more professional way. Her husband is an industrial research chemist, who is presently working on carcinogenesis in the industrial environment. He had originally helped June in her business when he was between jobs. However, once he had taken up his present post June was left running the business on her own. The business was fully off the ground by December 1984.

One evening in February 1985 when she was alone in the house not feeling terribly well, to her horror she passed a large amount of blood and bloodclots in her urine. She had had a very difficult winter and knew there was something wrong with her health although she couldn't quite put a name to it. She immediately phoned her daughter who instructed her to save a specimen next time she passed water and if there was still anything there to phone her back immediately. Things were just as bad the next time and so Lynda came and telephoned the doctor on call. He instructed June to go along to the Health Clinic the following morning with a sample of her urine. Her own doctor, Dr Harris, immediately made an appointment for her to see a surgeon, Mr Char, at Neath General Hospital.

After some outpatient investigations which were negative she was brought into hospital in March to have the cystoscopy performed by Mr Char. Thinking back to her meeting with the surgeon after this operation she says, "He was a lovely chap but I'll never forget it, it was like a scene out of one of those soap operas. I knew it couldn't have been good — he washed his hands so slowly and I thought — come on man, say whatever it is". He came around to the side of the bed, looked at me and told me that I had an ulcer with roots. Well — ulcer with roots I thought, that sounds pretty fishy to me. I said, "Is it cancer?", and he said, "I don't like the word", "Well is it?" I said, "Yes", he said, it was. "You'll have to have a big operation to have your bladder out followed by x-ray treatment", he said. "Well", I replied, "I'm not. I believe in spirit healing." "You've got to have more than faith to get rid of that", he said. I told him, "You don't understand; there's rays you know nothing about. You can keep your rays!"

"Well, he just looked at me horrified that I was refusing the operation. I was equally horrified that an operation was necessary. 'What am I going to do without my bladder?' I thought. No, the operation was not on. At that moment my biggest worry was for my daughter who worked in the same hospital. I was worried that she'd find out through the grape vine about this awkward woman with cancer who was going on about her special rays. I knew how upset she'd be to hear the diagnosis. I was more worried about that than having the damn thing!" Lynda having been summoned to come to see her mother, was reassured by her that she was completely confident, she could get rid of the thing on her own. "Come on" she said, "get a taxi — we're going home."

That was on a Friday. The following Tuesday she came to the Bristol Cancer Help Centre. June had heard about it from a friend in nursing and had also seen the programmes on television, presumably "The Gentle Way with Cancer" series. One of the sisters on her ward had also mentioned it: so all roads seemed to point to Bristol now that she had set herself so determinedly on her self-healing path. She told the receptionist at the Centre that she was "running away from the surgeons", and so she needed an urgent appointment.

Meanwhile poor Mr Char had decided to refer June to a Urologist; three weeks later she was asked to go and see Mr Vaughton at Morriston Hospital. When she received the appointment she thought, "Here we go, another fight". She did go along, however, and was told that the only treatment she could have was surgery as she had already had her full allowable quota of radiation when she had previously been treated for an ovarian tumour. June had been completely unaware at that time that she was being treated for cancer. "It was all a big fib," she says. "They told me that they were giving it to me because the ovarian cyst they were removing was full of pus and that it had burst — I needed the ray treatment to clear it up. I didn't think I'd be lied to, but there we are, those days it was all hush hush wasn't it? Don't tell her, she'll die of fright, that sort of thing."

Later she had realised that something was being witheld from her, but she still didn't know it was cancer. She became more suspicious as she realised that her doctors were increasingly surprised to see her continually coming back for check ups and she kept trying to have a peek at her notes. She was discharged after five years, as by this time she had entered the 'good prognostic group'. She puts her excellent recovery from her ovarian cancer down to the fact that she was having healing continuously through the early period of her illness. She believes that because the expectation is that you will only live for a short time anyway, the longer term side effects of the radiation treatment are ignored in favour of short term gain. She's sure the thinking was 'give her a massive dose now and she'll have five years'. She is sure now in retrospect that no one involved in her case expected her 'to get over all that lot'. She is utterly sure in herself intuitively that her bladder cancer is a second primary caused by the previous radiation treatment. She thinks that if she had known her diagnosis at the time and that if she'd known as much then about healing as she knows now that she would probably not have had the radiotherapy, relying on healing instead to clear up any stray cancer cells.

She did see Mr Vaughton who repeated the cystoscopy in April 1985 as mentioned previously. He confirmed the findings of Mr Char, and, knowing of June's resistance to an operation, tried to remove what he could of the tumour through the cystoscope. When she saw him post-op he again tried to persuade her to have the full operation, but she told him of her trip to Bristol and of her determination to do things her way. She said, "There is another way round this thing with alternative medicine you know, and I'm going to kill it dead. It's only three weeks since I had the diagnosis. It will take me three months." "Well," he said, "at least you're positive." She recalls, "He really looked worried, the poor man". When I asked, "What's frightening you then?", he didn't reply. I answered for him: "Frightened it's going to grow aren't you? Well it's not going to do that", I said, and headed for the door. I turned around and looked at him thinking, "Now I've done it, I've sent my parting shot, but perhaps I'd better hedge my bets a bit". "Should it grow," I said, "how will I know?" "You'll know", he said, "I'll see you in two months". "Good man", I thought, "so we haven't quarrelled, he'll still see me".

June was aware that to do the operation he had done was risky in its own right, as to remove the tumour partially could hasten its spread, but then she felt if she hadn't wanted his care and attention she shouldn't have gone to see him in the first place. As it turned out she had done the right thing. At the next interview with June following her third cystoscopy, Mr Vaughton affectionately welcomed her, saying "Come in black sheep!" He was as delighted as she was to be able to tell her that there was hardly anything there any more. He did still offer her a partial removal of the bladder, but June refused. She had had her three months to work on it and she had done it. All cystoscopies since that time have shown the bladder to be healed and healthy with only a small scar where the tumour once was.

Whilst shopping in Neath during the summer of 1987 June bumped into Mr Char. He asked her how she was. She teased him saying, "Those magic rays are working". She feels very affectionate towards both her consultants, describing them both as humble men, not the big 'I am' type. She says that, despite how difficult a patient she was she felt Mr Vaughton to be one hundred per cent behind her at all times, although she's sure that he found her rather frightening! She also says that she was really delighted by their generosity of spirit, as they were over the moon about her healing and were able to congratulate her rather than being caught up in their need to do it their own way.

## June's healing ability

Both June's mother and her grandmother were clairvoyant and June found that she had inherited their abilities. As an adult she felt that she wished to share her clairvoyance with others within a religious setting and she was thus drawn to the Christian Spiritualist Church. She has developed her ability to heal since joining the church. This happened after another clairvoyant at the church told her she was a healer, and so, in her own words, she just got up and did it. She has found that when she becomes ill her clairvoyant faculty dims. At the time of her ovarian tumour she had three teenage children, a mother with senile dementia to look after and the "radium trots" — that didn't leave much space for psychic phenomena! This is exactly what Katherina Collins said about the losing of her psychic faculty when she was so ill. Both feel that the denser states of mind associated with worry, illness and fear cause the loss of the fine tuning necessary to pick up psychic input. However, despite June's losing her clairvoyance at these times, she has retained her healing powers throughout both of her major illnesses; she is sure that as she returns to full health it is likely that "the gift of clairvoyance will be given back".

She feels that this is, "Because the power to heal is based on really feeling for someone and reaching out to them with your heart because you want to help them so much. The purer and stronger your intention, the easier it is to see what is really the matter with someone and the easier it is to heal them." In other words she may have temporarily lost her "fine tuning" but she never lost her compassion. She firmly believes that love is all there is. That it is all that we bring into the world and all that we take out again, and all there is in between is just so much material nonsense. While acknowledging that nonetheless we must have our feet firmly rooted on the earth in our material reality she also feels that we must never lose sight of its illusory nature.

Previously, when her clairvoyant powers were greater she could tell, using this faculty, whether people needed healing or not. Now she says that she can feel it through her hands. She says that she can actually feel a person's pain and tell them exactly what it's like; she can also feel it when the pain starts to come out of their body as she is giving them healing. She prays before she starts healing and asks for the power to be given to her. She strongly asserts that it is not her power but God's; for this reason she never charges for her healing. People are often so grateful that they try to press presents upon her: she especially loved the time when a little boy whom she had healed said to her, "What can I give you? — Want a brandy? — Want a chip?"

There are different types of healing, she says. She describes one type, which is quite distinct from the type of healing she practises, as "magnetic healing". It is dependent upon the individual energy of the healer; June says that she does not have this sort of energy to give out, and is in fact rather low on it herself, as shown by her tendency to become ill. However she says that if you work through the spirit you don't have to use your own energy. In fact, she says that she is always refreshed herself by healing because of the passage of the healing spirit through her, and jokes, "It always leaves a little bit behind". She also describes the notion of splitting the healing intention into different coloured rays dependent upon the type of condition being treated. She describes red, blue, pink, gold and green rays and how different they feel to give and to receive: for example some will be felt as hot or warm and others as cold. She does not have to decide what to do, but feels that instruction comes from healing guides: she is just the instrument. She says that what fundamentally happens, whichever type of healing is used, is that a person requiring healing is put into a state of ease. This often results in people falling into a deep sleep while receiving healing, especially if they are very ill.

She can use her own healing faculty on herself, and says this happens when her healing guide is with her. Remarkably she knows he is present by a sign in the form of a physical sensation she gets at the corner of her mouth, "as if a pen line had been drawn down from the corner of my mouth towards my chin". When her guide is with her she automatically goes into a state of deep breathing and relaxation. Nobody ever taught her this, it just comes naturally. She says that we all have our guides and that the guides of different healers work in different ways: this is why different people have fantastic results with one healer and feel absolutely nothing with another. She considers it important that the guides, patient and healer are in tune or are harmonious with each other or very little benefit will be felt. She would therefore encourage people to be discriminative in their choice of healer, trusting their feelings if they don't feel anything is happening. She would advise people to keep looking until they find someone who does make them feel better. The healer, too, would be able to tell you if he or she felt that healing was taking place. At the simplest level what is taking place is the giving of unconditional love which, if it is received, allows a person to relax and remove the armour of tension and anxiety which are formed by constantly trying to survive in a situation of real or imagined threat. Therefore in order for it to work, it is important that all beings involved, spirit or incarnate, are at ease with each other.

I felt impelled to ask June why she had come to Bristol at all when she was so incredibly confident about her own healing powers. To this she replied that she is not arrogant enough to think that she knows everything and felt there would be much to learn at Bristol. Certainly she knew nothing about the dietary and supplementation side of the Bristol approach and has found that she is far stronger physically on the diet. She kept strictly to the diet for four months, but has now adapted it to suit herself. She has also begun to cut down her vitamins, having taken the full regime for a year. She now finds that she can sense when she needs a boost of a certain vitamin, or when she's overdoing it. She is very aware of the fluctuation of her health in relation to her emotional state. However she has an interesting way of coping with stress: if she feels that her mental state is sufficiently bad that it is dragging her down physically, she does what she refers to as "going down into first gear". She explains this as mentally withdrawing into herself, becoming emotionally blank. She goes about her business in this state, only refocussing herself mentally if she absolutely has to. Another way she describes it is that she imagines how she would feel if she'd taken painkillers or tranquilisers and makes herself feel and act like it! In this state she will not rise to stimuli or situations which might normally make her blood boil. Again, therefore, relaxation was not new to her when she came to Bristol as she had already worked out her own technique, and neither was meditation, as this forms part of her religious practice.

Counselling was new to June, however, and has helped her to feel that she knows herself far better. The main result of this has been that she now takes much better care of herself; previously, she feels, she was doing a lot of "loving of her neighbours" without "loving herself", resulting in her having become very run down. This now means that she is better at drawing boundaries so that she does not make herself so constantly available to others; she will now only do so much before pulling back, or leave people to fight their own fights a bit more. Trying to be everything to everyone, she feels, was a result of a very poor self-image caused by a strict Welsh background. Her childhood was spent in the Welsh Valleys during the thirties, the depression years. Parents were much stricter with their children then and she had to 'mind her P's and Q's, and not step out of line'; June, being extremely sensitive, reacted badly to this environment. Instead of learning how to assert herself she learned how to please everybody in order to keep the peace. This is really what she is trying to change. She says of the approach, you can't completely change yourself, all you really have to do is alter enough to survive! She tries now, as a token of her new attitude towards herself, to spend a little bit of money on herself rather than always spending on her family, and she has also even managed to re-upholster some of her own furniture! She is definitely not returning to upholstery professionally as she feels this was too heavy for her, contributing to the breakdown of her health.

Another aspect of the Bristol therapy which was new to her was imaging. She used to image a fish swimming around her bladder taking big chunks of her tumour away. She also used to shed light on her tumour as she believes that no tumour can stand healing light. While she was using these images she would also imagine white corpuscles clustering around her bladder, breaking down the tumour and taking it away.

June believes that there is a purpose to suffering, and believes in the concepts of reincarnation and karma. She recalls a conversation with a healer friend: he said to her, "You know that you arranged all this for yourself before you were born don't you?" To which her reply was, "Yes well, I must have been twp".(Welsh for daft.) He went on to say that to her the purpose of her illness has been to help others by being living proof of the power of the divine. For all her jests she does believe in the idea of elective suffering. She thinks that it's all preplanned and that life is a test which enables us to learn more and more about our true natures. However she does not feel that elective suffering is equal to passive acceptance of fate.

She asserts that she once actively changed 'fate': she had once been told by another clairvoyant that her brother would die before her mother. She assured this man that this would not be the case, with as much conviction as she told Mr Vaughton that her cancer would not grow. Many months later when she had almost completely forgotten this meeting she spent a whole day feeling ghastly and very edgy. The following morning she awoke feeling even worse. She knew that she must contact either her brother or her son but had no idea why. She is certain that she did not consciously remember the message she had been given all those months before.

She had the feeling that the timing was crucial, and was "jumping around like a cat on hot tiles" waiting to make the call. When she finally made it her brother was really annoyed because she had caught him on his way out of the front door; still, she kept him chatting for a few minutes with nothing of importance to say. He was steadily growing more annoyed. Then came the moment when she "just knew" it was now all right for him to go. Later, she learned that on his way to work that morning he was three cars behind a very serious car crash. "Of course," she admits, "this proves nothing". However the premonition of her friend has not come true as her mother has since died. This of course is a very extreme example of the application of intuition and will. In the main she would just say that you have to be positive and fight your own fight. "The cancer was my fight," she says, "all anybody could do was help me".

She is so certain about the cause of her bladder cancer that I was intrigued to know what insight she had about her first cancer. She is sure that it was caused by her move from her home town, Aberfan, where she had lived all her life, to the Neath area. This move was caused by the lack of work in Aberfan. She could see the sense of the move and was quite positive about it but found once she got to Neath that she felt completely isolated and estranged in her new environment. She had young children and was therefore virtually housebound; she had no friends or relatives living locally to support her, and gradually over the months, "went into a decline". She knew she was ill and tried to convince doctors for four years that something was wrong with her. She had chronic discomfort in her abdomen and was convinced that she needed an operation. She said that in the end she was so desperate that if she'd had a mirror and a knife she would have done it herself! This is a very funny paradox considering how hard she has fought this time not to have medical treatment.

June is certain that spiritual healing and medicine can go hand in hand. She sees no reason whatsoever why there couldn't be healing rooms within hospitals. She feels then that patients could have the choice as to whether or not to use this facility. However she feels that people do have to want healing in order to open themselves to it, and therefore would never suggest it as a routine procedure. She would like to acknowledge her own healers, Mr Yorrie Morgan who called on her three times a week while she was ill, Mrs Pearl and the other healers from her church, and Mr Peter Short with his 'red ray'. June remembers Pearl saying to her at the crucial moment, "You will not have to have your bladder removed, in a short time you will be laughing about it". She now says with all the loving support she received from her healers and surgeons, how could she fail to get well?

In summary then, June's faith and spiritual awareness were so strong already that she only needed Bristol to bring the mental and physical aspects of herself into balance.

On death she says, "What's there to be frightened about dying? You've been there before. So OK, I just didn't want to take the early train home — I didn't like the colour of the ticket this time."

She is deeply grateful to her doctors for respecting her wishes and not continually undermining her by forcing their views upon her. Her ultimate accolade to her doctors is that she was able to have the best of both worlds: she was able to have orthodox and complementary treatment. Her orthodox doctors were able to meet her dependency needs as well as being generous enough to tolerate her belief system. Her message to all fellow 'doormats' is, "Do not let people take you for granted. A favour is a favour and certainly not a right." And to all of us she says, "Rely upon yourself. How you react is important. What is handed out to you is beyond your control but how you react is not. Do not let your problems get you down. Remember that whatever your problem is, it is not worth getting cancer for."

## Chapter 7

# Mary Carr
## Medical History

*Submitted by Dr M.H. Cullen, Consultant Medical Oncologist, and Dr D. Nixon, General Practitioner.*

Mary first presented to Dr Nixon in March 1982 complaining of a chest pain that she had had for some time, but which had become much worse, causing her to make the appointment. There were no abnormal clinical signs. However, the following month she presented with breathlessness and signs consistent with superior vena caval obstruction (SVC). He sent her immediately to see Dr Cullen at the Queen Elizabeth Hospital, Birmingham. Chest x-rays showed a right paratracheal mass. Mediastinoscopy was performed and biopsies were taken from the right paratracheal region. These turned out to be extensively infiltrated with anaplastic carcinoma. The cell population was mixed, consisting of some small anaplastic cells as well as large cell anaplastic carcinoma. Abdominal ultrasound and all blood tests were found to be normal. As these tests failed to reveal evidence of tumour in any other part of the body the lung lesion was presumed to be the primary. It was felt that the best chance for success was to treat her as for small cell anaplastic carcinoma with combination chemotherapy and mediastinal irradiation. Prior to commencing treatment Dr Cullen explained in detail the diagnosis, treatment and likely side-effects. He added that the prospects for permanent cure were slight (but definite), but that the chances of remission and prolongation of survival were quite good.

Chemotherapy was commenced on May 13th, consisting of intravenous Cyclophosphamide, Adriamycin and Vincristine. The SVC obstruction resolved promptly and mediastinal radiotherapy was commenced. She had a total of six courses of chemotherapy in all with steady objective regression of her tumour. Unfortunately, she was left with quite badly scarred lungs as a result of the radiotherapy. Treatment was discontinued in September 1982 and she has remained in clinical and radiological remission ever since. She is still underweight for her height.

## Dr Nixon's Comments

At the time of writing Dr Nixon says that Mary seems 'extraordinarily well' and that despite being somewhat limited by her breathlessness, she is fit and active and has returned to teaching. He feels that her prognosis at presentation was extremely poor, and that statistically her chances of survival must have been less than 1%. Now, over five years on, he feels this view must be changed; although one could never regard her as 'cured', the prognosis now has to be regarded as good. Despite acknowledging that "someone has to be in that lucky 1%", he acknowledges the role Mary has played in beating her disease, and says that her case has reinforced his feeling that however gloomy the prognosis, one should always be able to hold out some hope of cure. His general policy on the giving of prognosis/diagnosis to cancer patients is to be as honest as possible with due regard to the patient's own wishes, and to a lesser extent those of their relatives.

## Dr Cullen's Comments

The vast majority of patients with anaplastic carcinoma of the bronchus who are not cured with treatment relapse and die within two years of diagnosis. Since this patient has now survived five years since treatment commenced the prospects for long term survival ('cure') are now very good.

## Mary's Story

Mary's story is rather different from her doctors' comments. She feels that while her medical treatment saved her life when she was critically ill, it, alone, did not heal or cure her of her cancer. Going back to early 1982 she remembers that she had been feeling unwell for some months and had been to her GP two or three times. Her symptoms had been fairly non-specific and no diagnosis was made. She had felt palpitations and very odd pains in the centre of her chest, but an E.C.G. (heart tracing) had revealed no abnormality. Initially she experienced stabbing pains, and later just a dull ache. It appeared to Mary that her symptoms were stress related; certainly all her symptoms were worse with acute stress and in general she was going through an extremely unhappy period of her life. Mary had thought she was going to be found to have high blood pressure as she had suffered from this during her pregnancies. She has wondered whether she actually influenced the GP into confirming the diagnosis of stress and not looking any further for physical abnormalities, as she was so convinced that it was the cause of her problems.

At a later stage a new GP who was a respiratory expert joined the practice, and as the pain was still grinding on, he was brought in to offer an opinion. He, too, found absolutely nothing and thought that in view of her stress she should have a short course of valium (sedative medication). By this time she was getting much more suspicious. She didn't feel that valium was the answer and never took it. She remembers thinking at the time, "If this man says there's nothing wrong with me I'm going to go straight out of here and get myself the biggest life insurance policy I can find". She knew intuitively that it was only a matter of time until the whole thing came to a head, and within a few days of that consultation she became acutely ill and was rushed into hospital. Suddenly the veins in her neck had blown up and were standing out like ropes. She could hardly breath. Initial x-rays revealed nothing abnormal. She thinks that nobody really considered the possibility of cancer to start with because she didn't smoke and was relatively young. She then underwent tests for TB, thyroid problems and clots on the lung. When all these proved negative she was transferred to the cancer hospital in Birmingham.

It was at this point that Mary began to panic. It was established that the blood flow to the heart was being impeded by a mass pressing on the main vein carrying blood back to the heart from the head. There was a brief theory that the mass was due to Hodgkins disease. This diagnosis allowed a fair degree of optimism about the treatability of her condition. However, after the bronchoscopy, her husband was asked to come in so that they could be seen together: from this Mary knew that the diagnosis was going to be very bad. The mass had turned out to be lung cancer. She asked Dr Cullen directly what her chances were. He side stepped the question saying that that was immaterial and that he would treat her anyway. She realised from his reluctance to discuss any hopeful statistics or give her any encouragement that her prognosis was very poor indeed; that she possibly had months rather than years to live. She says, "I was suddenly so ill that I really didn't want to know exactly what was happening to me. Within a week I had gone from being a normal person to being someone who was terminally ill and had to be wheeled around in a wheel chair because I was too breathless to walk."

Mary is now very grateful that Dr Cullen didn't give her an exact prognosis. She thought at the time that she had about a thirty per cent chance of survival, and while she felt that thirty per cent was fairly daunting there was still a chance. She now realises just how poor her chances really were and thinks that if she had been given the full picture at that time she would have been too defeated to even embark upon a constructive programme.

She is full of praise for Dr Cullen's positive approach. He immediately concentrated on what could be done, offering to treat her with chemotherapy and radiotherapy. At the time she took this to mean that there was quite a good chance of a cure as she believed that due to the expense of the treatment, had he felt the situation to be hopeless, he would not have offered her anything. Her chemotherapy involved six three-weekly courses of the drugs mentioned above and ten treatments with radiotherapy. At that stage she could do nothing for herself as the treatment made her so ill that most of the time she was flat on her back. However, this treatment did get her to the point where she was able to breathe normally again.

She says that initially she was in a complete state of shock. She was sure she was dying and for the first few weeks was amazed each morning to find she was still alive! She can remember giving her husband David exact instructions on how to bring up their three children who were 5, 8 and 9 at that stage. Mary was entirely dependent on the help of her husband and her children's teachers, who, she says all gave unfailing support. David was a tower of strength at all times and genuinely convinced her throughout the course of her illness that he had complete faith she was going to be all right. Her mother, too, was convinced that Mary would survive. She had consulted a doctor friend who had said that Mary's chances were one in a hundred. Her mother replied without hesitation that Mary would be that one. A girlfriend who was told that Mary would not survive, was also completely convinced that this was not true. All this positivity was extremely helpful to Mary and gave a huge boost to her flagging confidence.

Towards the end of her treatment Mary heard about the Cancer Help Centre from the local methodist minister's wife, Grace Parry. She told Mary that the night she had heard the diagnosis she was completely unable to sleep, and during the sleepless hours she had felt 'directed' to help Mary. She therefore promptly got hold of, and brought Mary literature from the Centre. What particularly appealed to Mary in what she read was that here was something she could do for herself — she did not have to remain a passive victim of her situation, continually having things done for and to her. All other aspects of the programme made sense to her too, so she decided to do what she could at home until she was well enough to go to Bristol. She felt that the diet was a very important symbol of her intention to live even if it would not be curative per se, and so she started it straight away. David was a great support, making gallons of carrot juice for her as well as getting her vitamins and minerals organised. He also got her the Simontons' book on imaging and meditation, and she took up these practices all by herself. Grace's next idea was that a support group should meet regularly at Mary's home. This consisted of Grace and her husband, Dan Parry; another vicar and his wife, Freda and Bob Horsfield; and a teacher friend, Ivy Griffiths and, of course, David. The power of this group to restore Mary's hope was immense.

Mary began to feel satisfied that she was really doing something towards healing herself although she did find it extremely difficult to maintain concentration during imaging or meditation. She believed that the Bristol regime could not cure her but could give her the strength and tools with which to begin to fight. She did have faith that somewhere inside herself she had the power to get rid of the disease.

An extraordinary part of Mary's story was the visit of an

evangelical Christian who is clairvoyant, who was very worried about a 'presence' in her house. He felt that it would help if this spirit was laid to rest. Mary and her family knew that they had a ghost in their house, but had stopped thinking about it as they felt no tangible ill effects. (There was a theory in the village that this ghost was that of the old clock maker of Cleobury Mortimer.) The exorcism was duly performed by the local vicar with immediate results. All ghostly phenomena ceased from that day onwards. Mary has no strong feelings either way about the significance of this in her overall healing but mentioned it as another unusual thing which happened while she was in the process of fighting for her life.

She also received some healing from an evangelical minister which was most helpful to her. On one occasion his visit 'accidentally' followed that of one of the GPs from the local practice. He was late and the GP was early so the order of their visits was reversed. Mary had developed some neurological (nerve) symptoms after one of her chemotherapy sessions and the GP raised the possibility of brain secondaries as a possible cause. By the time he left Mary was completely devastated. She felt she could just about cope with lung cancer, but the thought of brain cancer defeated her altogether. By the time the minister left however, she felt much better in the 'knowledge' that this was a temporary set back caused by the chemotherapy. It turned out that she was right.

She says that once she was 'out of the woods' the minister told her that when he first came he was pretty daunted. She was bedridden then as she was only able to take two steps at a time without having to stop to rest. After forcing herself to do a little more each day she got across the landing and back. Then she managed to get downstairs. After that it was circuits round the dining room table followed by a trip to the end of the garden and back. It was a big triumph for Mary when she actually crossed the road and went to her friends for a coffee and even better when she got herself to the shop down the road. The minister said to Mary, "When you first invited me to come I was expecting you to need a few prayers — not a complete miracle!"

Mary had arrived at some sort of status quo until one day, soon after the treatment had finished, she received a visit from her own GP, Dr Nixon. It was September 23rd, Mary's mother's birthday. Dr Nixon had received a letter from the hospital which he felt he had to discuss with her. It said that she had now had all the treatment she could have and that sadly her tumour, although smaller, was not gone altogether. All that could really be done for Mary now was to provide her with lots of 'tender loving care'. It was obvious that Dr Nixon really did think the end was nigh, and they even talked about where Mary would like to die.

When David got home he immediately contacted Dr Cullen for verification of this dreadful news. Dr Cullen suggested they came to see him as soon as possible. He was very kind and positive but did not refute what had been said in the letter. He stressed to Mary that the most important thing was that she didn't think she was dying. Although she clung to this hope, the implication of this letter hit her like a sledge hammer. This was the first point at which the whole thing had really sunk in, and the fear of dying gripped her completely. She realised immediately that despite having been on a self-help path for months, she had not even begun. She realised it was now or never. The fact that orthodox medicine had done all it could and that she was now completely on her own brought everything into focus. Whatever perceptual filters she had managed to maintain to protect her from fully appreciating her situation had disappeared in one fell swoop.

Fortunately the medical treatment and her own determination had got her well enough to visit Bristol for an appointment. She needed to rethink her whole situation and make sense of what was really going on. What emerged from her discussions on that first visit was that during her imaging and meditation she would always get to a certain point and then fall asleep. She realised that in the context of her image what was happening was that she was symbolically allowing herself to die every time she fell asleep. She had repeatedly just given up the struggle. She now had to have the ultimate reckoning with herself — did she really want to live or did she actually subconsciously want to die. She realised that she had been saying that she wanted to live and had been going through the motions of trying to get herself well, but that underneath this was not really the case. She now believes that this is very common among ill people. She went home from Bristol and entered into a nightmarish two week confrontation with herself from which she emerged exhausted but triumphant. She had chosen life.

She then began with superhuman effort to perceive what her body needed to be well. One thing she remembers is that she was convinced that she should maintain all her concentration on her body and on wanting to live. She would not even allow herself to read, feeling that if she lost concentration for a minute then her body would die. She says, "I couldn't afford the luxury of reading and letting my body kill me while my mind was doing something else". She feels that after the decision had really been made she changed gear completely. The imaging and meditation became easy, having seemed nearly impossible until that point. At home she intensified all her own self-help practices. Her healing group continued to meet frequently in her house but now she was able to be much more receptive. In addition to giving her direct healing they would also ask her what she would specifically like them to pray for, what thoughts she would like to concentrate on and what practical help they could give her. The group obviously subscribed to the idea that she was the expert on herself and would know the areas in which she needed the most support. This group was a huge help as it gave regular, structured input with which to back up her own efforts. They continued to meet for about nine months until she was completely through the crisis.

What is startling about Mary's story is that within a few days of this enormous realisation she began to re-experience the funny pains she had had in her chest leading up to the illness. It was a dull ache at what she now knew was the site of the tumour. It lasted for about four days, and Mary feared the worst. David tried to reassure her that exactly the opposite might be the case, and that the tumour could be shrinking rather than growing. She was to find out the truth six weeks later as she had to go back to the hospital for a routine check up. She says that first one set of x-rays was taken which was 'routine', then another set was taken, which didn't alarm her too much as they sometimes did take two sets, but when they took a third set she became really worried. She was horrified, thinking that this must mean that the tumour had gone completely beserk. She shakily entered the consultant's room. Here she was told that the reason they had taken so many X-rays was that they had been unable to find the tumour and they now felt confident having looked for the tumour from every possible angle to say that it had gone altogether.

She obviously cannot say exactly what caused her healing. The implication from Dr Cullen's summary of her case is that she was put into remission by his treatment, but Mary does not feel that it was as simple as that. She believes that her survival is nothing short of a miracle. Dr Nixon is also amazed every time he sees her to find that she is still alive. She completely acknowledges the role her medical treatment played in the management of her case, but feels strongly that it was only one part of her cure. She also believes that the honesty of Dr Nixon probably saved her life.

Mary says that ever since the happy day that she was told that she was completely clear of cancer the quality of her life has been quite different. She now takes great pleasure in every moment of every day. She says, "There is no such thing as a bad Monday any more — I am always so grateful to be alive". Another way in which she had changed is in her ability to let go of anxiety. She describes herself formerly as a real worrier — the type who would seriously worry about things which were completely beyond her control, as well as all her personal and family worries. She says that now she is far more accepting and only gets involved with things which are essential, and which she can do something about. Her old self sees this as rather callous and selfish, but her new self can see that what this means is that she is actually a lot more effective. She no longer wastes so much energy on trivia and on being depressed about things which are beyond her power to resolve. She says that now her priority is to have a positive effect on things she can change, rather than being miserable about not being able to make major changes in the world around her.

This state of positivity has not been transient for Mary. It would be easy to imagine that once the threat was past, the old thought and behaviour patterns would re-establish themselves but that has not happened to her, nor to any of the other patients I have met who have undergone a profound trans-formation. It is interesting that she sometimes feels that the cancer is growing again. When this happens she immediately intensifies her imaging, and to date she had always brought any symptoms back under control in this way. She is now so confident in her ability to do this that she says she doesn't even get frightened any more when it happens.

Mary feels that she took to Bristol like a duck to water.

Everything said there struck chords in her. She feels that they teach survival and the right way to live and she feels privileged to be able to teach what she has learned to her children. She was particularly grateful to meet other cancer patients who had managed to rid themselves of the disease. She says that it was the combination of the support she got from Bristol, her family and the friends, and the unfailing rock-like support of her husband and children which was so vital, and got her through the critical time. She also acknowledges the kindness of Dr Nixon, who called far more often than was 'necessary', and the cheerfulness and friendliness of Doreen Raynor, the Health Visitor. Friends appeared, some of whom came from the other side of the country, to take over the running of the house for a week or so at a time. Flowers, cakes, cards and letters poured in from well-wishers and prayers were said for her in many churches. The kindness of all these people inspired her to live. She says that she was reminded of Tinkerbell — with all those people believing in her existence she just couldn't die! She tells of the arrival on her doorstep one evening of a small boy with a bunch of herbs in his hands who said, "My Mum says you must have these for your tea". She duly took her herbs. Life was breathed into Mary by this and many other gestures of love that she received in those dreadful months.

Of all the therapies she engaged in, Mary feels that the ones which had the most profound effect were meditation and imaging. She tells the story of going out to dinner one night after learning these techniques wearing a sleeveless summer dress. She felt rather cold, was covered in goose-pimples, and could see that all the hairs on her arms were standing up on end. She was worried that her hostess would see that she was cold and feel embarrassed, so she told her body that it wasn't cold and immediately the goose-pimples vanished. She says if you think about the efficacy of that trivial example of the influence of the mind on the body, and then multiply it up in proportion to the amount of time, concentration and mental determination exerted if your life is at stake, you can easily believe in the possibility of imaging your cancer away.

Mary used the classic image of white cells gobbling up a nasty black mass of tumour. This did not change after her showdown with herself. She says, "It was me that was wrong, not the image". She has never used the transformative type of imagery.

She kept absolutely rigidly to the diet for three years. Her family still eat a wholefood diet and this is really one of the only remaining outer signs of the enormous change which Mary underwent. Inside she feels completely different. Mary is quite convinced that the acute cause of her illness was stress and a recent bereavement. Two years before the onset of her illness her father had died. This hit Mary very hard indeed as her relationship with him was complicated and unresolved. Her move to Cleobury Mortimer had also proved very traumatic at this stressful time and she feels that this combination on top of her chronic unhappiness had eroded her will to live and triggered her cancer. Mary did find it important to think about and find a cause for her cancer as she felt that if she understood how it came, she could do more about getting rid of it. She cannot go as far as some of the patients and actually say she's glad she had cancer, as she has been left with so much scarring of her lungs that she is now somewhat disabled — a heavy price to pay for self realisation. On the positive side though, she says that she now knows herself better than ever before and also has far greater insight into the behaviour of others. She is much better at picking up subtle personality qualities and at sensing the difference between true motivation and motivation based on self deception or purely the avoidance of emotional pain. She also feels she has learned the difference between the relevant and the irrelevant in her life and relationships. She is now far more discriminating and as a result lives a much happier, fuller existence.

## Dr Cullen's views on the Centre

Dr Cullen's general view of the Centre is based upon reports from patients of his who have attended and from a thorough examination of literature and tapes that these patients have been given by the Centre. He feels that Mary has clearly done very well, but there is no doubt that a minority of patients with lung cancer can be cured with chemotherapy and radiotherapy without any alternative therapies. He says that in Mary's case it is impossible to evaluate the effect (if any) of the alternative therapies offered in Bristol. He can report however that her attitude to medical treatment was not prejudiced by her attendances in Bristol and that he feels in general that the supportive elements of the approach and the counselling offered to patients can be helpful. He would prefer this were routinely available within the N.H.S. His only worry in Mary's case was that he feels that the diet interfered with normal weight gain after her illness. Patients of his have reported the diet to be unpalatable, but he is happy that the nutritional content per se is usually adequate.

Other patients of his who have attended the Centre have not fared as well as Mary. He feels that there is no doubt that some feel great pressure not to 'cheat' as far as the diet is concerned and he is worried that because of the great importance attached to the diet in Bristol, any deviation can lead to major feelings of guilt and depression, particularly if this is associated with an exacerbation of the disease. This, he feels, is all the more worrying since "claims for the efficacy of the diet and meta-bolic supplements are not founded in properly conducted scientific trials". As far as he is aware, there is no evidence of the type generally required by practising oncologists that dietary and metabolic treatments of the sort offered in Bristol are beneficial. Indeed he is aware of evidence that a number of the metabolic therapies suggested are inactive and occasionally harmful.

Dr Cullen is bothered by the fact that the point is made in the Centre's literature that the success of the approach depends more or less exclusively on the patient's ability to make major changes in their attitude and diet. He feels that cancer patients are at a time in their lives when they are possibly least able to do this. He feels that the approach causes patients to blame themselves for their relapses or deterioration, when in truth he feels these to be a function of the illness itself, which in his view could not have been prevented voluntarily. He believes that there is a real risk that the Centre's approach can alienate patients from their relatives and doctors by "insisting that they should continue with treatment suggested even if relatives and doctors feel the opposite", and he is also concerned that the Centre risks undermining conventional medicine.

The technique of imaging the tumour and internal defences is in his view typical of many alternative therapies in that "it is surrounded by an air of mystery, is virtually impossible to evelute in scientific terms, and is not based upon any theories which are consistent with natural laws".

Possibly his major concern is "the implication from some alternative therapists that cancer can be caused by unsatisfactory realtionships". He says that one patient of his who attended the Centre "was led to believe that her breast cancer was caused by an unsatisfatory relationship with her father". This, he feels, is "simply untrue, and again can threaten relationships within families at a time when they need to be strengthened".

Dr Cullen is pleased that attempts are being made to evaluate properly the activities of the Bristol Cancer Help Centre in collaboration with a conventional oncology unit, and he looks forward to seeing the results of these investigations in due course. However, he is worried because "patients who attend centres like Bristol, and particularly those who continue to attend (the minority), are a highly self-selected group and so prospective comparisons are likely to be difficult and fraught with potential hazards". He very much hopes that these problems will be overcome and that the research work will be conducted promptly and reliably. He realises quite clearly that patients feel a need for alternative approaches to cancer, and feels this must be a reflection of the current state of conventional medicine in this country. His long term hope is that treatments of cancer should be scientifically tested and available to all within the N.H.S. In summary he says that, "Management should be conducted and treatment administered by properly trained professionals within the Health Service with care, sensitivity and skill".

# Dr Nixon's view of the Centre's Approach

Dr Nixon feels that all of his patients who have attended the Centre have been helped. He encourages patients to pursue any avenue of treatment they feel is right for them, but would always strongly recommend that whatever else they do, they should not ignore the medical treatment offered. He is far from convinced that the metabolic treatment offered at the Centre has any place in the treatment of cancer, although he admits that he has not read any papers which prove the issue one way or the other and has never seen this therapy do any harm. He does

believe that the progress of physical disease can be altered by
mental attitude and emotional state, believing that patients like
Mary who find the strength and support to fight their disease
may well alter their prognosis. He therefore condones the
Centre's practices which help patients to improve their mental
state; changing fear, hopelessness, and impotence to confidence, optimism and security.

*Chapter 8*

# Veronica Mills

Medical History

(*Birth Date*: 6 April 1942)

*Submitted by Dr Gardner (GP).*

Veronica attended Dr Gardner's surgery in December 1982 with a growth on the left side of her neck. She was referred to a physician, Dr Smith, and was diagnosed as having a malignant melanoma. She was referred to Mr Barry Corps, a plastic surgeon, who excised the melanoma in December, 1982. A CAT scan was then performed to check the rest of the body for the presence of secondaries. The result was positive, revealing a secondary melanoma in the right lobe of the liver. She was seen again in March 1983 by Mr Corps to discuss this finding. He informed Veronica that she had an extremely poor prognosis and that her life expectancy was in all probability around three months. He was unable to offer any further surgical treatment. He also felt that radiotherapy or chemotherapy were inadvisable as they would seriously impair the quality of what little life she had left and could not be relied upon to improve her chances. Veronica returned to Dr Gardner to discuss her situation. He supported her attendance at the Bristol Cancer Help Centre, deciding that, in view of her poor prognosis, he would give her his full support if she tried this or any other alternative treatment.

## Dr Gardner's Views

Dr Gardner feels that Veronica's visits to the Centre have helped her tremendously, especially from the psychological point of view. He reports that four years on she is obviously very well and very fit. He feels he cannot give an opinion about the general use of vitamins and minerals in the treatment of cancer patients, but thinks they appear to have worked in this case. He suggests that the success of the Centre's approach depends upon the patient's personality, predicting that only certain people will benefit, and says that he would exercise discrimination in referring people to the Centre just as he would in the recommending of radiotherapy or chemotherapy. He also thinks that good motivation and the full support of the family and GP are essential. He goes so far as to say that they are pre-requisites for success. He is very grateful to have learned about the Centre's existence through this case, and feels that patients cannot lose anything and may gain a lot from the Centre's approach.

## Mr Corps's Views

Mr Corps was most pleased to hear that the Centre is in the process of setting up scientific trials to investigate its methods. However he describes himself as extremely biased. While he accepts that the few patients he knows who have attended the Centre have been helped psychologically, he feels that the claims made by patients and the media about the relationship between diet and cure are 'utter garbage'. He says that he would perhaps not feel so strongly if the claims were not made in such extravagant and ridiculous terms. He has not written off all alternative therapy, as he admits he has known patients who have benefitted from spinal manipulation (albeit with dubious anatomical explanation of the treatment by the osteopath). He has no specific comments to make on Veronica's case as he has not seen her for over three years.

## Veronica's Story

Veronica and her husband Bill moved to their present house in Newcastle-under-Lyme in 1979. This move became necessary because Bill's employers wanted him to be based from the Potteries. Before that they had been in Bedfordshire for seven years and before that in Scotland for five. These moves, too, had been work-related. Veronica is originally from Luton in Bedfordshire, which is where she met Bill. She worked then as the secretary to the airport commandant at Luton airport, a fascinating job which she loved. They married in 1965. Three years later Bill heard that he had to move to Scotland and while Veronica was sad to lose her job she felt that this would be a natural break in her career which would allow her to start having children. They had decided right from day one that they wanted to have a family of four. So sure were they of this fact that on the plane home after their honeymoon they actually named their four children. They'd thought that they would leave it five years, but their posting to Scotland seemed to provide the ideal opportunity to start their family a little earlier.

After several months had passed and Veronica had still not conceived, alarm bells began to ring. They went off for fertility tests and discovered to their enormous dismay that they would never be able to have children. They decided immediately that the answer was to adopt. They had to undergo a very prolonged assessment period to confirm their suitability as adoptive parents. Veronica says it was a nightmare because it seemed as if where she was living there was a new baby born every week. All she could see everywhere were mothers and babies, and her time dragged by, with just the interminable spot checks from social workers and health visitors to look forward to. Even when they were finally accepted they were told that it could well be another two years before a child would be given to them, so she felt she must get a job or she would go out of her mind. She worked six weeks for the DHSS, an experience which she hated. She was feeling very vulnerable at the time, and didn't feel welcomed by the other women in the office at all. She felt they treated her like an alien because she was English. So she moved to work for a fashion company as a typist. She didn't want any responsibility at that stage, which is why she took this job but the management spotted her ability immediately and within a very short time she was made a junior executive.

Four months into this job she received a phonecall from Bill at work one morning. He said to her, "Are you sitting down?" She said, "No", and he said, "Well, sit down please". She could tell it was good news but never in her wildest dreams imagined it would be what she most wanted to hear in the world. "I'm coming to pick you up," he said, "we're going to fetch our baby daughter". Veronica just shrieked with joy. Tears were streaming down her face. She was laughing and crying at the same time. No-one in the office had the slightest clue what was going on. She hadn't confided in anyone because she didn't want to be treated specially in any way. This sudden arrival threw them into absolute turmoil because they hadn't even got a nappy, let alone a cot or any of the other baby paraphenalia but it was the happiest chaos imaginable. They named their daughter Tracey-Ann.

The next decision was to buy property, now that they had a child. So the upheaval continued for a few months longer as they packed up and moved. When Tracey-Ann was 10 months old they decided that it was time they placed their 'order' with the adoption society for a second child, in view of the potential two year wait. This time they waited a year and a month for the arrival of Alisdair, their equally precious son. If it had been possible they would have gone on to adopt two more children, but the rules of the adoption society were that after having two babies they would have to adopt an older child. They felt that this would be too disruptive of the overall family dynamic, and decided that they were more than satisfied with the two they had.

In 1973 the news came through that Bill was no longer needed in Scotland and that he would either have to leave the firm or go back to Bedfordshire. As work was rather thin on the ground in Scotland it seemed far wiser to go back South than risk unemployment. They bought a house in Ampthill, Bedfordshire. The big advantage of this move was that they were near their families again. The next seven years were extremely happy. Veronica formed some good, supportive relationships with other women that she met through the children's nurseries and schools and as a result some very special friendships developed. She became thoroughly integrated into the local community, chairing the local play group committee, and playing competitive badminton for the local club. It came as a very hard blow to Veronica then, in 1979, when the move to Staffordshire became inevitable.

Bill had been commuting up there a few days a week for about two years, so he had some good friends in the area already. The children were 7 and 9 by this stage, and their school was directly across the road from their new house. This meant that Veronica didn't even have to escort them there in the mornings. There was no easy way for Veronica to develop any sense that she belonged in her new environment, and after having been so busy, involved and relied upon in her old setting, she became very withdrawn and unhappy. To make things worse, funds weren't really available initially to redecorate to her taste, so for about a year after the move she felt like she was living in someone else's house. The result was that she didn't feel comfortable in the house nor in the neighbourhood. In Ampthill they had lived at the end of a cul-de-sac. There were always children playing outside, and she couldn't walk down the road without someone talking to her. Her new house was in a quieter, more suburban area. Privacy seemed to be the order of the day, and certainly nobody seemed to need anything from anybody else (or if they did they certainly wouldn't ask for it). So she wouldn't see a soul from the time the children left until they got home for tea. It was not for lack of trying, either. She made many forays out, and attempted to get involved with one group and another, but nothing stuck and certainly no new relationships formed.

The effect of all this was that she just couldn't think of it as home. Luton was still home, and she kept trying to get back up there at weekends whenever she could. She didn't feel able to express any of this to Bill because there was nothing he could do about it, and she didn't want to make him feel guilty. The turning point came one weekend when she was visiting friends in Hertfordshire. She was having a cream tea with her old next door neighbour, Linda. Linda suddenly turned to her and said, "What on earth is the matter with you Veronica?" Veronica was extremely taken aback and replied with some irritation, "What do you mean, what's the matter with me?" Linda was brutally honest. She told Veronica that she had totally changed since leaving Ampthill. She was now completely boring, had no conversation at all and seemed to be doing nothing whatsoever with her life. Veronica was furious, especially as Linda was so much younger than her. She felt that she ought to be the one having the insights and laying down the law about what was going on. Underneath, though, she knew Linda was absolutely right, and so the dam broke and she told Linda what was happening. Linda told her that when she went home she must immediately find some work — stacking shelves in a supermarket if necessary — anything to get her out of the house and talking to people again.

The reason Veronica hadn't considered working again was

because she wanted to be there for the children after school, and anyway she had got out of the habit of thinking about working while she was occupied full time with the children during their infancy. As she contemplated looking for work she realised just how far inside herself she had sunk because the thought of being out of the house in a shop or office terrified her. She sat at home on the Monday morning after that weekend, having packed Bill and the children off to work and school, and wept into her morning coffee. Linda was absolutely right. Her life was a nothing. Outside her role as Bill's wife and the children's mother there was a complete vacuum. She was very depressed. The other thing which was very hard for Veronica was that she was going through a premature menopause. This had started when she was 35, three years before leaving Ampthill. She'd had to have an ovarian cyst removed and the surgeons ended up taking away the best part of both ovaries. They had hoped this would not precipitate menopause, but soon after the operation she started getting all the symptoms. Her skin changed, becoming blotchy and more wrinkled, she got terrible hot flushes, but worst of all her sex drive disappeared completely. She felt so unattractive and 'freakish' that she couldn't even contemplate the idea. She hadn't really received any good medical support over this, and this contributed heavily to her depression.

One of Linda's suggestions had been that she apply to Marks and Spencer to do Christmas work. So after she had recovered a little from her desperation she plucked up enough courage to phone them. To her amazement she was called for interview, and to her even greater amazement she got the job. She did two half days per week in the men's wear department during the five weeks leading up to Christmas 1981 and was delighted with the whole set-up. She loved the activity and social contact, and was extremely happy when the firm asked her if she would stay on after Christmas. They only asked five of the forty Christmas temps to stay, so this gave her confidence a big boost too. She'd rather forgotten at that stage what an excellent track record she had, and how efficient she is. Bill was only too happy to accommodate her needs and came home early when she was going to be back too late to be there for the children. She suddenly felt so emancipated. She finally had some time and space which was her own. Because of her office skills she was asked once or twice to help out when they were short staffed, and predictably it wasn't long before her potential was spotted and she was asked to move into the office. This was a little disappointing because of losing the social part of the job, but she accepted because with it came the chance of an extra half day a week. The other encouraging development that year was that she found a new GP, Dr Gardner, and he managed to get her to a menopause clinic in Birmingham for specialist help. The main boost from that first consultation was that she discovered how common the phenomenon of premature menopause is, which meant to her that she was therefore not a freak after all. Perhaps even more important, though, was that a doctor took her problem seriously and made her feel cared for. This enabled her to come to terms with and accept her state much better, and of course from that point on nothing seemed so bad.

It was during a routine visit to Dr Gardner in the December of 1982 to get a repeat prescription for her menopause medication (prescribed by Birmingham) that she mentioned in passing that she had a funny lumpy mole on her chin. She always used to fiddle with it affectionately when she was sitting doing nothing, but had realised that it seemed to be getting slightly bigger. It wasn't painful or itchy, but she just wanted him to have a look anyway. He remained completely calm and collected and just said, "I'm not sure, but we'll have it off anyway". She groaned and said, "Not this side of Christmas please, I've got so much on, I can't cope with any extra hassle". She went back home and thought nothing more of it. The very same day the receptionist from the surgery phoned to give her an appointment on the Friday of that week with a specialist. She was rather taken aback, having specifically asked if she could wait until after Christmas, but said if they had gone to that much trouble to get her the appointment of course she'd go. She duly set off to see the specialist, entirely ignorant of the possible complications. After taking her history, he calmly announced that he would ask sister to get a side theatre ready and that he would take it off there and then. She said to him that that was awfully kind of him, but actually she was going to the school 'Hoe Down' that evening, thanked him very much, but said she'd come another day!

At that point he looked very uneasy and said he really must insist that she stay and let him do the little operation. There would only be a few stitches anyway and he'd make it almost invisible. At this point she was beginning to become suspicious. She asked him straight out why everybody was in such a damned hurry. He said it was because there was just a possibility that it was malignant. Nothing like this had even remotely occurred to Veronica. She was instantly reduced to a state of trembling silence. She obediently went and sat in the waiting room while they prepared the theatre. Bill couldn't be reached on the phone, and there was no-one else locally to whom she was close enough to ring for emergency moral support.

The doctor quickly and efficiently removed the lump. Veronica asked to see 'the creature'. She says it looked like a peach stone with all the little fibres hanging from it. Of course, it looked much bigger than it was because it was in fluid by this time. When he had finished he said he'd be getting in touch with Mr Barry Corps to see her. Still reeling from the first shock she said, "And who is Mr Corps?" "Oh, a plastic surgeon", he said. Veronica clutched at her chin, "What have you done to me", she gasped, "Why do I need a plastic surgeon?" "Nothing, nothing", he said, pulling her hand away from her fresh wound. "It's just that if it is malignant we'll have to clear the whole area. But don't you fret, I'll arrange the whole thing." "Fret," she said, "I can't even engage my brain". She felt that he paid no attention to her at all, just to the lump in the jar. Now she is absolutely amazed at the way that she meekly went along with everything she was told to do, without asking for more explanation, time, or at least the chance to get someone she knew to come and help her through the ordeal.

He left the theatre and she remained there, hanging on to the sister, whose poor hand must have been practically bloodless by this point. She was wonderful. Veronica was crying hysterically, shaking like a leaf and completely unable to move. Her stomach was churning and she felt physically sick. The nurse stayed with her until she was steady enough to talk, then got her home phone number. By this time Bill was home and came rushing down. At this stage she was still lying in the operating theatre as she had been too weak to move. Between sobs she tried to explain to him what had happened. She gradually calmed down, and eventually was able to let Bill take her home. They sat and talked the subject round and round in circles, and finally she decided that the best possible thing for them to do after all was to go to the school dance!

She still can't quite believe she did it. But she calmly got herself ready and off they went. She said, "It is like when you hear that someone has died, after the initial shock you get a strange sense of inner strength". In all moments of complete crisis during her illness she has had this sense — as if she has tapped into a completely different part of her psyche which just knew what to do.

A week later she and Bill went for the results, to be told that the lump was a malignant melanoma. The next hurdle was that she had to face major surgery to clear the whole area around the original lump. Mr Corps explained that he would need to remove an area of skin approximately four by two inches, and that he would then cover this area with a skin graft from another area where the pigmentation matched best. He explained exactly how he would make the incisions and that the graft site would be the worse of the two injuries. She says, "I was quite sane by this point. We discussed all this as if it was an engineering project. I had got used to the idea that this had to be done and had accepted it. Again, totally naively, it never occured to me that this would not be the end of it. I just took it for granted that that was all I would have to go through. I didn't look any further. I had never even heard of secondaries. I didn't know what a secondary was, and had no indication at all that there was any possibility of this."

She went in for her operation on December 27th and came out of hospital on New Year's Day of 1983. Bill's mother came for three weeks to help them over the worst of the aftermath. Veronica was somewhat mystified when she came round from the operation because, after having had all the elaborate explanation and warning about the skin graft, she could find nowhere on her body where any skin had been removed. The other thing that had just slipped past her without her giving it a second thought was that she had been given a total body scan the day before her operation. She accepted that this was part of the routine pre-operative work-up procedure.

She is extremely thankful now that she didn't know what they were looking for, because she thinks she would have been sick with fright. When Mr Corps came round he said that the reason she hadn't had to have a graft was that he had been able to move the skin around the wound enough to cover the defect, and that the scan had been clear, so all was well. She went home and as far as she was concerned it was just a matter of getting well. She was cosseted by Bill's mother and the family, and she just relaxed and soaked up all their loving care.

Six weeks later she was called back for a 'repeat routine scan'. She thought of this as the final all-clear routine before the file was closed for ever. However this time it took ages for the results to come through. She was aware enough of what was going on to know that the technicians see whatever they see there and then. It wasn't as if anything had to be processed, or await specialist comment. So she thought this was all rather suspect. She phoned Mr Corps's secretary after two weeks had passed, who said she couldn't read it out because she didn't really understand it. Veronica said to her, "Come on, I'm not a child, if you're saying that there's something on there you're not prepared to tell me please will you give me an urgent appointment with Mr Corps". She was asked to come up that afternoon. This time, as Bill was out on the road, her next door neighbour said he would take her. He had heard the story of the first incident and didn't want Veronica to be alone. She tried to dissuade him, saying she'd probably have to wait ages, but he insisted.

She went in to Mr Corps's room. She sat on one side of the desk and he sat on the other. She apologised for jumping the queue, but said she had had to come because she feared the news was bad as she hadn't heard anything. He shook his head and said she was right — the news wasn't good. She asked him what he meant and he said she had a secondary. She says, "I then had to ask him what a secondary was, that's how stupid I was". He explained that it was more cancer, but that this time it was in her liver. She gasped and said, "Oh crikey, I've only got one liver! You can't remove that can you?" He confirmed that this was quite true. She asked him what else he could do about it, to which he replied that really there was nothing at all he could offer her. He said that he had discussed it with his oncologist colleagues, and that they had decided that as she was actually quite well and feeling no ill effects from this tumour they would not treat her at all, because the treatment would make her feel so unwell and most likely make no difference at all to the outcome of her disease. At this point she asked the big question. "That's all very well," she said, "but if there's no treatment for me, how long does this mean I have to live?" She was feeling more and more unreal — as if she was actually in a horror film and not a doctor's consulting room. She says, "He looked at me, and his face was ashen. There was no movement in it at all. It was just like a screen. Then he just shook his head." She spluttered and stuttered, "Wh-wh-what do you mean? How long have I got to live?" He looked at her and said, "Months, — maybe three months".

At that moment all she wanted was some human contact. She wanted someone to hold her. His hands were tightly clasped together on the table, and she reached out and took hold of them, but they were absolutely locked in tension. She picked them up and shook them saying, "You can't tell me that, you can't tell me I'm going to die".

There had been a small defect in the liver on the first scan after all, which could only be confirmed now as a secondary because it was still there on the second scan but bigger. He reiterated everything he had said, adding that all she could really do now was to go home, contact her GP for support if she had any faith in him, and get the most out of what remaining life she had. This was not enough for Veronica. She still had hold of his hands but by now was banging them up and down on the table shouting, "You can't tell me I'm going to die". He was transfixed with horror and she was hysterical. She just wanted to get some feeling out of him — to have him come round the table and take hold of her, but he didn't. When it became completely clear that they were at an emotional impasse, she dragged herself to her feet and left the room. She put her head round the waiting room door and beckoned Arthur, her neighbour into the corridor. He said, "My God, what's wrong?" and she said, "He's just told me I'm dying, he says I've got to die". Arthur looked at her as if she was completely mad. He said, "Don't be so silly Veronica, you're perfectly all right, there's nothing wrong with you. You're not going to die." "Oh no Arthur," she said, "I've got an inoperable tumour of the liver and you have to die with those".

By this time they were walking down the steps. Arthur was just about able to keep her upright. When she got out into the street all her strength came flooding back. She started stamping her feet and screaming, "I am not going to die, I AM NOT GOING TO DIE!" Arthur held her and eventually managed to get her across the street saying all the time, "You're right, of course you're right. There's no way you're going to die." He got her into the car, did up her safety belt and drove her home. When they got there Veronica realised she couldn't go into the house as the two children and her mother were there. She was still hysterical, her skin had come out in big red blotches and she was an absolute mess. So Arthur took her into his house. His poor wife looked on horrified as he led Veronica to a chair. He poured her a very large brandy. By this point she says she was beginning to have the most extraordinary sensation she has ever had in her life. She says, "My whole body started to vibrate violently. It was nothing like trembling or anything you could get a hold of. I had lost all control. It was like a million volts going through me. I couldn't move and I couldn't speak. I thought I was going to explode or go completely insane."

In this peculiar state she noticed that there was a telephone beside her. Again what she calls her inner strength temporarily took over. She picked it up and phoned the GP's surgery. She said, "This is Veronica Mills. I've just been told that I'm going to die. I can feel the top of my head lifting off. I'm either going to lose my mind or explode. Please get something or someone to me immediately." Unfortunately Dr Gardner was right in the middle of his evening surgery so they asked her to send someone up to collect some tablets, and said that he would come as early as he could in the morning. Arthur left straight away for the surgery. A few minutes later Bill walked in. He rushed over and knelt down in front of her. She relived the whole experience with him. He just looked at her and said, "No Veronica, this is not happening to us. I don't believe a word of it". Meanwhile Arthur had got back with the Valium. She took one. She had had another brandy by then and was beginning to feel a bit more relaxed. By complete coincidence, they were supposed to be going to another dance that night — with Pat and Arthur. She laughs now, saying that those were the only two dances they had been invited to all year. To all of their amazement, she suddenly picked herself up and said, "Look at the time, I'd better go and get the tea ready". Pat said, "Whatever for?" And she said, "Have you forgotten, we're going to a dance?" Pat said, "Are you mad, we can't possibly go now that all this has happened". "Yes we can", said Veronica. "It's happening to me Pat, not you, and I say we go. I'm not dying today, I've got three

months — I'm not spoiling the night for anybody. Get your-
selves ready, we're going." And with that she left to go home to
face her mother and her children.

They had obviously realised by now that all was far from
well. Veronica calmly explained that Mummy's news had not
been good news, and that she had not been ready to hear it, so
she had been next door crying. She was all right now and
everything was going to be all right. The children accepted this
and got on with what they were doing. It was somewhat harder
for Veronica to comfort her Mother, though, because she had
lost her husband nine years previously, within three months of
his having had major surgery for his cancer. The next morning
the GP came as promised. He was extremely shocked as nobody
had communicated the information to him about her secondary
and dreadful prognosis. Veronica found this appalling. She says
she was really angry, even then, because she felt the least that
could have been done was to have alerted her GP as a safety net
to catch her after the blow had been delivered. After all, they
had known the result for two weeks when she was informed.
She says she would actually have much preferred to have been
told by her GP, because he knew her already and could have
taken far better care of her.

He was very kind to her and stressed that the first thing she
must do was to let go of the thought that she was dying or she
would 'die to order'. They talked about her shock, disillusion-
ment and disbelief at the fact that the first time she had had to
ask the 'all-powerful medical profession' for any help it had
nothing to offer her. They talked about the way her father had
died of cancer — slowly and painfully — and she conveyed to
him her horror of the possibility that she might have to die this
way. She also told him that there was no way she could die now
anyway because she couldn't desert her children at this stage.
She had fought so hard to get them. She couldn't possibly leave
them yet. She still had 'a job of work to do' — namely their
upbringing. He eventually managed to calm her down, and his
parting words as he left the house were "Watch the telly tonight,
there's a programme on about a place in Bristol that's got a new
approach to cancer".

She says now, "God does work in some mysterious ways you
know, that was the first of the series of six programmes on the
Centre". The turn-around that that programme caused for her

was extraordinary. She had spent twenty-four hours in complete and utter desperation, and suddenly after watching that programme she was 'not a doomed human anymore' — there was something she could do after all. Bill was in Bristol the next day and called in to pick up the tapes and literature. She couldn't actually get there for six weeks though, because there was such a rush of bookings after the first programme. So she started on her own because six weeks was half way through the three months she had been given. Although she got on with the diet and tapes to the best of her ability, she says that before she got to Bristol she was 'still dying'. She knows this was how she really felt because she got in her vicar, David Marsh, for a crash course on preparing to die. She had ignored her spiritual practices for a long time and felt the need to tune in again rapidly. She felt that if she died she would be meeting God, and she was far from ready to do that. She also realised from the literature that counselling was important, so she knew the next task was to find herself a psychologist.

Dr Gardner was very helpful and said that he would be quite happy to prescribe the vitamins and minerals recommended in the Centre literature if she could find out the details. Yet more support was to come from a pharmacist called Peter Taylor, who by complete coincidence, she had been seated next to at dinner on the evening she received her dreadful news. She contacted him with the details of what she needed and he immediately made it his business to get Veronica the very best quality vitamins on the N.H.S. The 'coincidence' was not to stop there. The same day she went round to his house to discuss what she needed, there happened to be a district nurse there who was looking after his mother-in-law. She pricked up her ears at their conversation, and said she knew someone who had been to Bristol. Veronica assumed it was another patient, but the nurse said no, he was a psychologist who had gone to study the approach. This turned out to be John Hegarty, who became Veronica's counsellor and who has since set up a counselling service which is available through the N.H.S. to all cancer patients attending the North Staffordshire Royal Infirmary. His own interest had been triggered through losing his mother with cancer. Veronica and he developed an excellent relationship and did some very deep work together.

Veronica says that initially "he completely carried me". He

allowed her to offload all her fears about her cancer and death. This quickly led them into the area of her overall fearfulness and poor self-image. Another problem for Veronica was in the expressing of love and affection. She also discovered how much grief she was carrying over the loss of her father. She realised how little she had known him during her life. It was therefore a great comfort to her when a spiritualist told her that her father was very much with her. She now thinks of him as God's messenger whom He has appointed to look after her and get her well. In this way she now experiences a love and comfort for and from him that she was never able to have while he was alive. She often talks to him as she is driving along in the car. In fact she uses her car itself as a bit of a therapy centre. She may sing, shout, relax or commune as the mood takes her.

John and Veronica argued fiercely about two issues. One was that she refused to accept that she was dying. The second was whether or not she should tell the children that she was dying. This she absolutely would not do. It was too negative for her. She says he may even have been playing Devil's advocate, because it all actually served to strengthen her resolve in these areas rather than weaken it or undermine her. She feels that over the months she shed layers and layers of superfluous defences, fear and tension, until eventually it was obvious that this process had reached a natural conclusion. He left it up to her to come to him if she needed him, and she rings him "if she needs to scream". She says that she returns from her visits feeling thoroughly cleansed. She hasn't needed to do this for a year now. It became less necessary as she mastered the techniques of meditation and relaxation. John also helped her with visualisation, and got her to draw some of her visualisations for them to work on together, which was extremely helpful. She says that the counselling was far from easy. It was really gruelling work, dredging up all her old pains. She'd had no idea that there were so many childhood hurts and sadnesses there under the surface, clogging her up.

After a couple of months Veronica began to realise that most of their social contact had dropped off. Even the family seemed a bit 'thin on the ground'. So one night Bill, realising that this was because they were all so frightened and embarrassed, drew up a big list of all their friends and relatives and phoned every single one of them. He told them all the exact details. Yes, she did have cancer, and yes, she had been given three months to live. But they were fighting it in every way they knew how, and they needed support. He asked them all to look for and read anything they could which might help, and to keep the information coming. He and Veronica were not frightened to talk about it, in fact needed to talk about it, so would they all please draw closer and not retreat into the distance. Veronica said it was quite incredible. After feeling as if she was on an island, the love and support and ideas just started pouring in.

When she and Bill finally got to Bristol the main thing they wanted was to meet someone 'who had done it'. In their terms at that time this meant someone who had outlived their prognosis. They wanted something tangible to hold on to. Initially they felt themselves to be very different from the people running the place — as if these people weren't really quite of this world. They therefore found it all a bit odd, but say this was quickly compensated for by the feeling of love which emanated from everyone. They spent the happiest, safest-feeling day there that they had spent since the diagnosis had been made. They still remember how good it felt to laugh that day. It was as if they'd forgotten how. Now she cannot praise the staff of the Centre enough. She says they are extraordinary people. Nothing is too much trouble, they just keep on loving and supporting you whatever happens. She says, "There is no way I could have uncapped the healing potential in myself without them. They presented me with a treasure chest of ideas and things to do. They helped me open the lid and there were all these exciting avenues just waiting to be explored."

In those days patients were asked to complete psychological tests on arrival. When she went in to see Dr Alec Forbes after completing hers, he promptly told her that she was the kind of person who would be inclined to project what she thought other people wanted to see, and that there was no need for her to do this with him. This was very powerful for Veronica. She felt 'known' already and stripped naked of her defences. While this was rather frightening it was simultaneously a great relief. She found his dynamism and utter conviction in the rightness of what he was doing and suggesting extremely comforting. A lot of the subtler aspects of the approach went over their heads initially, but they said that they were just so grateful to have something to do, instead of sitting around waiting for things to take their course.

Veronica does think, in fact, that the Centre is rather unrealistic about the practicality of carrying out the approach if one has a family or is having to support oneself, because following the regime is a full time occupation. On the other hand, she knows that for many people it is necessary to fill all their time initially to keep themselves from thinking continually about dying. In her own case, she had to find a balance between giving herself the time and space she needed, and not scaring the children by suddenly completely changing her, and therefore their lifestyle. As the days had gone by it had come out that she had cancer. They knew you died from cancer, because their grandfather had. The only way she could cope with their fear was by keeping everything as normal as possible to prove to them that everything was all right.

In fact, the stark reality came out quite inadvertently one day when Veronica was asked to speak on the local radio. The children had rushed home from school to make a recording of the programme. The interviewer asked if she'd been given her life expectancy and without thinking she calmly said, "Oh yes, he gave me three months to live". When she got home Tracey-Ann was fine but Alisdair didn't appear. Veronica still didn't realise what she had done. So when he came down rather subdued, she asked him whatever was the matter. He said, "Did they really say you've got to die?" She immediately realised to her horror what had happened, and tried hard to reassure him. She said it was true, that was what the doctor had said, but that was months ago and look how well she was now. He just looked at her and said, "I've been thinking about it Mummy — no one knows when you're going to die". She picked him up, hugging him tightly and loving him more than ever said, "Alisdair, you're absolutely right, nobody knows when we are going to die!"

They came to love their visits to Bristol. She says in a way it was like going home to mother, as if she was crawling under a great big protective wing, for a little period of time, where she could be safe, protected and nurtured. The benefit of the Centre built up gradually for Veronica and Bill. There was no sudden transformation or release as for Reg and Evelyn; their confidence grew over the weeks. Initially they were inspired to keep up their efforts, helped greatly by seeing others who had done it, and very glad to have a structure to hang on to. As the weeks went by they were amazed to realise that they were now part of the group who had beaten their prognosis and were themselves inspiring others in the open forum meeting.

Dr Gardner coaxed her into celebrating her three months by having another body scan. Afterwards the radiologist came rushing over to her and said, "Have I got good news for you — somehow you've managed to contain your tumour!" Veronica almost leapt off the bed into his arms. She said, "I knew I could — and now I'll go and get rid of it altogether". She left the hospital in a state of euphoria. A woman in the street asked her if she had 5p for the phone. She looked in her purse and said, "Oh yes, here's one, oh and here's another, look I've got four in fact — please take them all!" She emptied her purse into the woman's hand and went on her way, grinning from ear to ear, leaving the woman standing there in dumb amazement. The next call was the surgery. She burst into Dr Gardner's room shouting, "We've done it, we've done it", and gave him a big hug. He was nearly as happy as she was.

This result gave her massive inspiration to go on with her self-healing efforts. Following her 'crash course' with the vicar, David Marsh, when she thought she was dying, she made the decision to carry on with her spiritual study and entered confirmation classes. She was confirmed in the November of 1983 by the Bishop of Stafford. This made a huge difference to her. In the course of this year she met a retired physician called Dr Christopher Woodard. He is a lay preacher and healer. Veronica found him enormously inspiring. He would sit and hold her hands and give her 'God's healing'. She said he exuded such energy, and would say to her, "You're not going to die. Just live — take your time and live". One time after she had seen him she can remember skipping up her drive. Arthur poked his head round the door and asked her what was happening. She told him, "It's all right Arthur, it's going to be all right — I can live". Three years later Dr Woodard spotted her in his congregation in a little country church. She had gone especially to hear him preach. Afterwards he found her and said, "I just couldn't help but look at you throughout the service, I knew your face and managed to place you finally — you are so alive. You've got nothing at all to worry about, God is within you —

your eyes say it — here I am *living*." When Veronica left that
church she felt as if she was walking on air. She says, "I can do
all sorts of things now I could never do before; I can think for
myself, I understand my body, I can change, and I can even
redirect pain, but I'm just like everybody else — I need constant
encouragement and that man was absolutely brilliant at it."

Veronica also set up weekly healing sessions for herself with
a woman healer nearby, and got help from an herbalist/
iridologist too. At this stage the Centre was still recommending
the use of coffee enemas. The rationale is that it is supposed to
help the body clear itself of toxins which have accumulated over
years of unhealthy eating. Her herbalist, Kitty Campion, who
is an expert on the bowel, advised Veronica that chicory root
was six times more effective than coffee, so she changed to
chicory and carried on with this practice for eight months. She
also prescribed all sorts of other cleansing and tonic remedies.
Her body felt wonderful after this time so she decided enough
was enough and she would stop the enemas. She has carried on
with a very healthy diet ever since her diagnosis. She will
occasionally eat cheese, fish and chicken, but is otherwise very
strict.

After a year Bill changed to the diet too. This was a great help
to Veronica because she was then far more inclined to make an
effort to make the food interesting. Her daughter also took to
the diet, but Alisdair's tastes have polarised in the other
direction, and he has actively chosen to be a 'junk food man'.
The family have openly discussed this and everyone respects his
choice. In fact at one point John Hegarty came and did a family
session with them all, because Bill and Veronica noticed that the
children were developing quite strong negative feelings about
her and her illness. So much of their parents' time and energy
had been devoted to keeping Veronica alive that the children
had taken something of a back seat. Understandably, they were
getting rather fed up and angry that Veronica's needs always
came first, both emotionally and financially. Alisdair pointed
out to her that it was OK if she wanted a new juicer — they
always had the money for that, but if he wanted a BMX bike
that was a different story. He has continued to use Veronica's
lifestyle and needs to create reactively his own stance and
attitudes. Veronica thinks he is all the stronger and better able
to express himself for this. Her daughter, on the other hand, has

reacted by constantly bending and accommodating like a willow. Veronica worries that she has picked up her own old way of always putting the needs of others first, and thinks that this situation has given her little opportunity to enjoy her childhood before clicking into 'responsible mode'. The family meeting therefore proved to be extremely useful. The facts of her situation were separated out from the fear and the fiction, resentments were expressed, and the meeting was really quite cautionary for Veronica and Bill as they realised that the children had more or less been parenting themselves for quite some time.

Veronica got on particularly well with imaging and meditation. She found very early on that once she got relaxed it was almost impossible for her to use the aggressive Simonton type of imaging. Instead, her main image in the early days was of a huge, swirling, purple cloud that would enter her body through the top of her head. This represented power coming 'from above'. The clouds were quite fluffy and light and would gently roll through her in flowing waves. The purple colour represents cleansing and purity for her. It is also a reassuring colour to her because it reminds her of bishop's robes. Sometimes the cloud would be blue rather than purple and occasionally it would have a vivid gold line around the edge of it. This always made her feel especially good, as if she'd got a gold star at school. Very occasionally the cloud would be green or yellow, especially if she'd been outside drawing energy from the sun.

She always directed the cloud through her whole body, as she says she never knew her tumour was in her liver until someone told her, so it could be anywhere. She often refers to her tumour as 'the creature'. She hasn't really given it a form, but says it would be relatively benign and not terribly ugly. She feels that while it is a potential aggressor, it has actually failed because it made itself visible, so she really doesn't think it is so very intelligent. She says that they live in symbiosis. They tolerate each other. They do not have any sympathy for each other but they both know the rules. If she 'goes to sleep on the job', he wakes up and talks back. This may take the form of an ache or general feeling of malaise. That in turn wakes her up again. She feels it is terribly important not to go into headlong battle with it because that only gives it power. She feels that if she'd gone in for radio- or chemotherapy then the creature would have gone in deeper and found somewhere quieter than her liver to live. She says, "If it stays put and doesn't trouble me why should I trouble it?" She also feels that fear gives it power, and that one of the major battles for the cancer patient is therefore to become free from fear.

During the October of 1983 she really had to put her new-found strength of mind to the test. After a particularly achey day she decided she'd feel her liver. She'd never really thought of doing this before. To her horror she found a big lump. It was so obvious that if it had been there for long she's sure she or one of the doctors would have noticed it. Dr Gardner came and said that it was either the initial tumour which had grown or a new tumour. She decided immediately that there was no way she was going to have any further medical tests; she would simply intensify her Bristol programme. The next cause for alarm was that she started losing weight rapidly. This terrified her as she knew this was often the beginning of the end. She was thrown into complete turmoil and started wracking her brain day and night in the hope of finding a stone she had left unturned.

Katherina was an enormous help to her, and began to teach her how to stop giving the tumour all her attention. She insisted that Veronica must forget it altogether and carry on as usual. She started replacing the totally negative thoughts she was having with thoughts like, "Why do I have to assume it's cancer? In fact how does anybody know that a blob on a scanner is cancer? It could just as easily be a cyst — after all I've had cysts on my ovaries — maybe I never had a melanoma of the liver after all." The other way she decided to look at it was that it was a healing crisis she was going through. She thought to herself this is the tumour in its death throes. It hadn't completely gone up to now because a sneaky little part of her still believed in it. She was still living as someone who should have been dead by then, so no wonder it was still around. It had woken up again to get her to go the whole way and drop it altogether. She says now the lovely thing is she can tell herself almost anything and believe it. In these, and many other ways, she relentlessly turned any signal she got from her mind and body into a positive rather than a negative. Everything that came up was an opportunity to learn and grow.

She had a bit of a struggle over meditation at this time too.

She felt that if she had no tumour, why did she need to do the meditation and imaging? Wasn't that just another way of acknowledging the presence of the tumour? She learned eventually to do her meditation "as an average human doing it for their well-being". She therefore used this overall crisis to help herself shift gear from focussing on finding a cure or battling to stay alive, into purely focussing on her total well-being. This was really the true point of transformation for Veronica.

She decided to join a meditation group locally which was not for ill people and found this tremendously helpful. She says that meditating in a group like this makes it much easier because of the feeling and energy that is generated. She describes the feeling she gets after meditating as "a freedom from all pressures, aggression or sadness, or a sense of great wellbeing and complete peace with the world". She often meditates for up to 45 minutes at a time, but would strongly recommend that everyone practises meditation for at least 15 minutes a day. She feels even this would change most peoples' experience of life for the better.

She used an imaging technique to help get rid of her worrying thoughts. Every time a difficult thought would arise she would image herself putting it into a box. If it was a minor one she would gift wrap it and put a big bow on the top, but if it was a horror she'd put it in a crate, nail the lid down and chuck it to the bottom of the ocean. She will admit however that there was a very fine line at that time between keeping and losing control of her mind, and at times, her sanity. She stresses that no-one must get the idea that this approach is easy. She says, "It would have been far easier to let go and be seduced by the fear and by death itself. At times it seems so much easier a path to take even for someone as awkward and determined as me." She says though, that once you have managed to crawl out from under the fear, the sense of liberation is quite heady and that if you really do practise meditation regularly these battles become far easier, and less and less frequent.

Dr Annie Pye at the Centre was also a source of great new inspiration. She asked Veronica if she'd ever considered acupuncture. She'd had a friend with leukaemia who had reversed a terrific weight loss with the help of acupuncture. So Veronica immediately sent for the Register of Acupuncturists for her area and chose Ian Hurley who was nearby in Hale. By coincidence, he turned out to be a good friend of Penny Brohn's. He took Veronica's problem extremely seriously and did a lot of research and study on how best to help her. Over the next 18 months they clawed back her lost stone and by the end of that period he said, "If you keep coming to me I'll be taking money under false pretences. Your body is balanced like a finely tuned engine. You are in perfect health."

One thing she did vow to herself after this nasty experience was that she would never go feeling for lumps and bumps again. She has still never felt the area to this day to see whether that lump is still there.

She has also derived great help from doing guided imagery. She sees her images as vividly as reality. She can now use the 'journeys' she has been taken on by the various guides at home on her own. She loves to visit a rose garden and go round drinking in the perfume. She always picks herself a yellow rose while she's there. Another favourite is to take herself up the side of a mountain. There is a path with tiny earth steps cut into it, supported by wooden boards to stop the steps from crumbling. The smallness of the steps means that there is very little effort involved. She is very excited and happy as she climbs up because she is going to visit a temple. At the top of the mountain around the corner she comes upon the temple. It is pure white against the blue sky, and has a white dome like Sacre Coeur. She knows that Christ is waiting inside for her. There are no other people there. Entering the church and coming into Christ's presence fills her with complete ecstatic joy.

Veronica, like Mary, says she can spot very easily the patients who will make it and the ones who won't, unless some radical change occurs. She says it's quite simple, you can just see who is really hungry for life and who isn't. The ones who aren't just make a token effort, or pay lip service to the approach to placate their relatives. For her there was no time lag or numb period while she waited to find the will to live. It was realer than real from the first moment she was given her diagnosis. Unlike Katherina and Mary, she didn't have to wait for something or someone to make her angry enough or determined enough to want to live. She knew she was going to fight it, and win, the minute she got out into the street from Mr Corps's consulting room. Her complete confidence in this fact and the inner strength she has tapped into have amazed her. The other thing that has astonished her is the number of 'coincidences' that have occurred since being on this path into the heart of life. Her vicar said to her, "They're not coincidences, they're God instances". It is remarkable how many people who come to Bristol report this same phenomenon of synchronicity. It seems that once people start to look for and ask for help, things start opening up all around them in the most uncanny but marvellous way. She feels that once you've been stimulated and really have the belief that you're not going to die, all the rest just comes. "I didn't actually have to search at all," she says, "everything just fell into place".

She often refers to "the new Veronica". I asked her what was so different about her now. She says she can easily sum it up by saying she's now alive. She feels far more confident, far more aware and far more complete. She says she now enjoys each and every day and says that this has been the biggest lesson — to live for the present. She says before she was moody and irritable and that has completely gone. "Before," she says, "I was Bill's wife. Now I'm Veronica Mills. Before I just blended in with the scenery. I just existed in the support role. Because of this tumour I now have a wonderful circle of friends. They are people who have really loved, supported and inspired me. It's as if the whole world has opened up to me. I'm not at all angry with this tumour. If it's taken this tumour to give me the fabulous life I have now, then I'm really grateful to it. It's as if I was on the wrong path. It took the tumour to bring me back to the crossroads and now I've chosen the right path. It was all there already. Nothing was put on this earth for me, it just took a tumour to wake me up to the richness and wonder of life."

Her husband agrees there is a big change. He says she's much more demanding and determined. Often people come back to Bristol saying that everyone around them thinks the new person is much less 'nice'. Once they stop putting everyone else's needs first, people get quite a shock. While Bill realises this is much better for her, he says that it's taken a lot of adjusting to. He says he quite often switches off, and occasionally rebels if he's feeling really brave! Bill doesn't share Veronica's new spiritual leanings either (although he is a Christian). Occasionally they both wonder if Veronica will keep growing at such a pace that she will either become so self-contained she won't want her marriage any more, or that they will become so different that they will cease to have enough in common to sustain a marriage. However they both feel this is unlikely as they have formed such a strong bond over this battle for her life.

As I talked to Bill he was surprised to realise to what degree the philosophy has rubbed off on him. For example, he thinks he too is much better at communicating now. He can talk far more freely about his feelings. The other thing he has noticed is how much his priorities have changed, and how odd other peoples' values seem. For example, at work he is amazed how much energy people put into trivia whilst missing the really important issues like caring for each other and the atmosphere and safety of the working environment. It makes it quite difficult for him at work because he's supposed to go in with the hard sell, and finds himself far more concerned with the person he's with and what their circumstances are. He is really considering leaving his job to find work with people. He doesn't necessarily mean in the caring professions, but any sort of work where he could treat people properly.

At the time I saw Veronica she had been declared entirely tumour-free by both her healer and her iridologist. Barbara (the healer) believes herself to be extremely sensitive to the presence of cancer and could feel it quite distinctly initially. She is now convinced that it has completely gone. These two therapists announced this independently of each other, which was all the more reassuring for Veronica. She has not been back to have this confirmed on scan because that seems irrelevant to her now. When she told Dr Gardner he just smiled and said, "Oh, fine". Veronica said, "Well, don't you want to know more?" He said, "Give it five years Veronica. When five years are up I'll be quite happy to assume it never happened." She sheepishly said to Barbara, "I believe you completely, but I don't feel quite ready to let go of seeing you yet". To which Barbara replied, "Oh no Veronica, I like to keep seeing people who've had cancer until they've been free for seven years". When I saw her she was bubbling over with enthusiasm, vigour and happiness. I too, from the overall impression she creates, would certainly find it very hard to believe she was still carrying any cancer.

Veronica is full of praise for her GP. "He is so tolerant", she says. "He has been a tower of support and has shared every stage of the adventure with me. He never criticised any of the steps I took and encouraged me all the way." She is also immensely grateful to her employers, Marks and Spencer. When she first had her diagnosis the manager of her branch actually came round to the house to ask if there was any way in which they could help. He asked her to stay away from work for a little while so that he could tell all the others. This would give them time to shed their tears and get used to the idea so they could treat her as normally as possible when she came back. In fact her work mates raised over a thousand pounds to support her in her alternative treatments. The head doctor from the central office in London travelled all the way up to meet her, and invited her to come up to London to visit him and tell him of her progress. He was fascinated by the approach she was taking and was very keen to learn from her. When she did go to London the firm treated her like royalty, entertaining her and showing her all around the central set-up.

When I asked Veronica which of the therapies she thought was responsible for her healing she answered without any hesitation that it has to be God's will. She feels that all the therapies, love and support she has received have opened her up to allow her spirit to shine through and that it is her spiritual fulfilment which has caused her body to fall into line. "After all," she says, "I am such a small inconsequential speck on the earth; How could I have brought this about myself? I'm just not strong enough." She says this does not mean that she's a born again Christian or an 'alleluyah type' that will stand about on street corners telling everybody else how to live their lives, but just that she knows now in every fibre of her being that if you truly ask for God's help and put yourself completely into his hands that all will be well. She recognises however that this is a dynamic partnership, and not just a question of sitting back in blind faith. She has found, though, by putting herself in this state of surrender and trust in God's love, that the work she had to do became obvious, and help and guidance has appeared at every step of the way.

Her comment to the medical profession is simple. If you close one door you must open another. To leave a person with no hope and nothing to try is tantamount to killing them. Veronica believes so strongly in the notion of medical gloom becoming a self-fulfilling prophecy that she is going to write a book of her own called 'Programmed To Die' in which she will try to express the intensity of her battle to overcome the shattering effect of being given her prognosis. She has to concede however that Mr Corps's honesty probably saved her life. If she hadn't been given such a shock she may never have mounted such a massive campaign of self-preservation.

## Author's Review. March 1989

The above chapter was written in the Spring of 1986. During the Winter of 1987, Veronica was suddenly overtaken by lung secondaries. She had remained extremely well up to that point, but developed a very certain sense that all was not well during November 1987. Return visits to the hospital for scans revealed that fluid was building up in her lungs and it became clear that the cancer had spread. The situation became more and more severe through the Spring of 1988, and she became fully aware that she was rapidly approaching death. She embraced this final illness with all of her characteristic courage, calm and awareness and died a fully 'conscious' death on the 27th May 1988.

Her husband spoke to me shortly after her death and told me he had never witnessed anything so perfect and beautiful. He watched Veronica grow and grow in emotional and spiritual stature as death approached and said that the quality of her presence in the final few days and hours was quite magnificent. Their relationship also grew to a peak of intensity previously unimaginable to Bill, and even now his grief is mixed in equal parts with the joy he still feels in his knowing and closeness to Veronica.

He has been kind enough to write about those final few months, and I have included the following piece in his own words. He adds, however, that no words can ever really express the state of joy and love that he experienced through the pure communion that Veronica and he achieved.

## Veronica's Final Illness, by her husband, Bill Mills

Following a considerable period of well-being, it was during November 1987 that Veronica discussed with me how she was feeling in her body. She said that she felt "ugly inside". This statement of fact was made with such conviction and awareness that we both understood the gravity of the period we were about to enter. We had reached a healing crisis that would be difficult to overcome. There was no question that we would change our approach or lifestyle with the arrival of this new problem. On the contrary: we had grown so much from similar crises in the past, we knew that walking hand in hand into the heart of these new difficulties would continue to improve our quality of life and increase still further our awareness and mutual spiritual commitment. In retrospect, it was as if we knew inwardly that we had now been launched on the 'programme' which would eventually culminate in her passing.

Up to the time of her death, Veronica and God became even closer. It was inherently obvious that they were side by side. There were so many hills to climb, obstacles to overcome and adjustments to be made, all of which were tackled with surprising ease. They had the appearance of happening in slow motion.

Her first visit to hospital was highly emotionally charged. We were both walking on broken glass, stepping back into the system which had rejected us five years previously. It was necessary for Veronica to take charge in this situation, cultivating people and tuning them to her spiritual level and way of thinking. It had been assumed by all we met that we would automatically accept any treatment they offered to us. However, at the outset we had made a pact that whatever future developments might bring, we would reject last ditch orthodox treatments in favour of 'quality of life'. Veronica wished to preserve her dignity. So when we entered the hospital this second time, this pact was to be put to the ultimate test. As the days passed, the protein-filled fluid round the lungs began to consolidate, making it harder and harder for her to breathe. We were required to call on all our resources. The strength of Veronica's character really showed through; her spiritual stamina came to her rescue. Rightly so, for it was at this time that the full and complete realisation came to the fore; there was to be no recovery from this state.

We shed floods of tears together. This was not because we had failed in our battle to keep Veronica alive; the tears were a mixture of happiness and sadness. We were sad because of the unknown territory into which we were to pass. We were happy because of our enormous sense of achievement. Veronica's now natural ability to hold the situation in proportion was helping all those who came into contact with her. The ward sister recalls that when looking into Veronica's eyes it was so obvious that it was Veronica that was helping her, rather than the other way round. This ability of Veronica's fully illustrates the height of awareness that existed within her.

By the time we left hospital, we were completely free of the fear of 'the ultimate'. An air of security radiated from Veronica. It was as if we had switched automatically into another phase of the programme; this time to undertake an extended farewell. Instinctively we knew how to behave towards each other — with confidence, awareness, love and devotion. Veronica's disabilities did not diminish our relationship. She would often remind me of her sexuality, bringing her womanhood to the fore. It was beautiful.

Spring was always her favourite time of the year, so it was fitting that she could spend the last weeks of her life in this season. Most of her time was spent in the garden where she would sit to receive a constant stream of visitors. Her welcome was as enthusiastic whatever the time of day. She paced herself to achieve this. People were so precious to her and she was precious to them. She had earned the respect of those around her which allowed them to give unconditionally. Throughout this period her spiritual development benefitted us all. She knew that people were coming to say their goodbyes and she made that easier, comforting and warming them; leaving a little of herself in everybody. She prepared us in no small way to cope with her passing and our own individual lives thereafter. Those same people speak of her continuing presence today. She was fortified by those privileged to be continually at her side. The days seemed so long, again as if in slow motion, which added an extra dimension to those closing weeks.

For ourselves, we spent each morning and evening alone. They were peaceful hours and so precious when I reflect today. The immense bond we had grew and grew in this last phase. I had the pleasure of taking over all her most intimate tasks, as she became progressively unable to do these herself. Her appearance was so important. She felt it was vital to present her beauty both inner and outer. She continued to dismiss the negative, turning it into the positive. It made these simple tasks acts of love.

With hindsight, it is clear that we both knew when the eve of her passing finally came, and that it was the right time for her to leave. Unprompted, we gathered as a family in our bedroom to bid our 'goodnights', these to be our last as a family. It was a happy warm occasion with us all conversing quite freely with each other. Later, Veronica and I lay side by side holding hands, and some time passed before she broke the silence. In doing so she delivered to me with complete conviction and without sadness an epitaph which will never be erased from my memory. She told me with absolute confidence that our lives together had been complete and totally fulfilling. She and her God knew that it was time to say these final words. She had been granted the strength, even at this late hour, to prepare us for her passing and to prepare the children and me for life afterwards without her. Her passing was truly a victory. Veronica did not suffer. Now when I reflect, I realise I have no fears, no remorse, nothing left unsaid, nothing left undone, no bitterness — just sweetness. I have no doubts in my mind where my dear Veronica is and who she is with. Her reunion with Christ and God is her just reward.

Following her funeral, I was privileged to be able to meet all her mourners. It truly amazed me at the time and still does, how Veronica had touched the hearts and minds of so many people, some of whom I had not met until that day. So many said with conviction that they clearly felt her presence at the service, which I view as being evidence of her strength of spirit: her life after passing. Even now, when attending church on a Sunday, I get butterflies in my stomach at the excitement of the closeness of her spirit. I now know how she was able to leave us with such a richness of her memory and love.

In closing, I leave you with the reminder that she never gave up. She said that "if you find the resources within your own energies, and if you find a faith, whatever it is that you believe in, then life is for us all. If you then live each day as a totally complete day, accepting that tomorrow will come and see yourself as equal to every other person, with or without disease, you can go forward without fear". She learned that life was not about cure, but about experience. If one can be well enough each and every day to enjoy that experience, then that in itself is completeness.

# PART 2

## Chapter 9

# The Mind and Cancer: Causation and Therapy

by MICHAEL WETZLER, M.D.

The idea that the mind can be involved in the development of cancer has a long and fascinating history. As early as the second century, the Greek medical authority Galen is reported to have observed that melancholic women are more prone to cancer than sanguine women. In 1701, the English physician Grendon emphasised the effect of "disasters of life as occasion much trouble and grief" on the development of cancer. Later that century in 1783, Burrows suggested that cancer is caused by "the uneasy passions of the mind with which the patient is affected for a long time that weaken the circulation of the blood and consequently thicken it".

Nunn, in 1822, in describing the growth of tumours of the breast, "attributed to emotional factors causative influences on the development of cancer" and Walshe also during the 1800's called attention to the "influence of mental misery, sudden reverse of fortune and habitual gloomings of temper on the disposition of carcinomatous matter". Paget in 1870 expressed his opinion that "deep mental distress is among the conditions favourable to the occurence of cancer".

In 1893 the first statistical study was performed by Snow. He reported that out of 250 patients with either cancer of the breast or uterus, 156 had suffered from "an immediately antecedent trouble — often in a very poignant form, such as loss of a near relative or exceedingly hard work and privation". It took another thirty-three years, however, before there was a further important study. This probably reflects the fact that major breakthroughs were occuring in the physical areas of medicine and surgery at that time and hence very little emphasis was being placed on psychosomatic medicine. In 1926, Elida Evans studied 100 cancer patients using Jungian in-depth psychotherapy and found that "a typical cancer patient had lost an important emotional relationship before the development of cancer and was unable to secure any effective outlet for his or her psychic energy".[1]

Within the last few decades however, a great deal of research has been done in an attempt to demonstrate or refute these ideas. The work can be divided into two major areas. The researching of:-

1. The associations between personality and the development of cancer.

2. The associations between stressful life events and cancer.

## The Cancer Personality Theories

David Kissen, a distinguished chest surgeon, looked at the personality profiles of patients with cancer and noticed that traits such as the inability to express their true emotions or 'get things off their chests' was more common in those who developed lung cancer.[2] Schmale and Iker were two other researchers who looked at women who developed cervical cancer. They found that a "hopeless, prone personality" or "situations of hopeless frustration with respect to irresolvable conflict" were good predictors of the existence of cervical cancer.[3]

A prospective study took place in the 1940's at the Johns Hopkins University using medical students.[4] Originally its focus was on psychological factors which might predict high blood pressure and coronary heart disease, but data was also accumulated which gave insight into psychological factors in cancer too. The statistics suggested that there were possibly predictable categories into which the people who later developed cancer seemed to fall. They tended to be rather lonely people without any close parental affiliation or those who had figuratively 'lost their parent'. A significant correlation has also been established between cancer diagnosis and extreme anger supression, especially in females under fifty.[5] In this study K.W. Pettingale describes a whole range of personality characteristics attributed to cancer patients including:-

1. inability to express hostile feelings,
2. rigidity,
3. impairment of self-awareness,
4. introspection,
5. a tendency to sacrifice self,
6. a tendency to self-blame and
7. a predisposition to experience hopelessness and despair; as well as
8. an overall tendency for cancer patients to be people who have very few outlets for emotional discharge of any sort.

However, the most definite finding was a significant association between the diagnosis of breast cancer and an 'abnormal' release of emotion, especially anger, in adult life. In most cases the 'abnormality' was an extreme supression of anger but the other extreme was excessive expression of anger. Considerable work has been done in this sphere by the American psychologist Lawrence LeShan.[6] He found that the lives of many cancer patients had the following points in common:-

1. Marked feelings of isolation, neglect and despair as a youth with ensuing difficulty in interpersonal relationships.
2. The development in early adulthood of a consuming interest in either a strong and meaningful relationship or a satisfying vocation, which became the centre of their life.
3. The loss of this relationship or role, resulting in despair and reactivating the painful feelings of childhood once again.
4. A characteristic bottling up of despair.

He adds that cancer patients may often be described as kind, sweet and benign, but that this sweetness may well be a mask they wear to conceal their feelings of anger, hurt and hostility. This, he feels, is mainly because they have the type of underlying personality structure which has always handled stress in this unhealthy way (paradoxically, as a self-protective mechanism). Ultimately this has created feelings of loneliness and hopelessness and of being helpless and trapped; feelings which are described over and over again in the research of 'cancer psychology'. Interestingly, this is also borne out by a study which looks at how well people do who already have the disease.[7] Steven Greer, now of the Royal Marsden, divided cancer patients into four groups based on their attitude to their disease. He discovered that of his four groups, the first two did significantly worse in terms of outlook than the latter two. The groups were:-

1. Those who take a hopeless/helpless view of their disease and are in many ways a victim of it.

2. Those who take a stoically accepting view of their disease, seeing it in a sense as a decree of fate.

3. Those who deny they even have the disease. Included amongst these are:
   a. Those who have had medical treatment and who consider themselves cured by it and deny that there is any further risk, and
   b. Those who deny there is anything wrong at all until they absolutely have to, thereby delaying their seeking medical advice. (This does not mean that people who present late do better in general terms, but only that deniers do better than people who have equally advanced disease from the above two categories.)

4. Those who accept their diagnosis and the gravity of the situation but who will not accept their prognosis and take active steps to fight their disease.

It does seem interesting, that in terms of length of survival those who practise denial often do as well as those who take their disease head on. Both approaches involve a fight in fact, but with different goals. Certainly, it is hard to do the Centre's normal type of counselling with those who practise denial and with these patients the role of the counsellor is far more supportive and geared towards the formation of coping strategies than helping the individual to look at their illness and its possible significance. It must be said however, that whereas the approach of group four can result in a great sense of peace and understanding, that of group three seems to involve a continual and rather exhausting battle. This is why the Centre tends to encourage facing illness directly.

There are certainly other studies that also suggest that the risk to those who have lost their raison d'etre is greater than for those who have meaningful lives.[8] Other studies confirm Dr

Greer's work in the finding that patients who have maximised the significance of their illness in some way seem to recover from it far better than those who have not.[9] A further study confirming this showed that combative females who showed a self-willed, self-determining attitude to their medical carers seemed to survive longer when suffering from terminal breast cancer than otherwise matched individuals who were complacent and accepting.[10]

Although these types of studies abound it is so difficult to make them scientifically watertight that none of the above results have been treated as conclusive by the scientific community. However, it does seem significant that there has been so much overlapping of results, and that extremely consistent themes have emerged from this line of study.

## Life Events and Cancer

Discussion of the idea of a cancer personality quite often leaves psychologists, doctors and patients feeling understandably uncomfortable, both because of the difficulty of establishing the theory and because of the implication that a sector of the population is at risk by their very nature. However almost everyone, either intuitively or through anecdotal evidence, will accept that there is some relationship between what happens to us and how our bodies function. Common are the stories of the death of an old person within weeks or months of their losing their spouse (although one epidemiological study has shown this to be untrue[11]), and most people have experienced the deterioration in their physical health if they are heart-broken or suffer a sudden shock.

Not only have studies shown an increased incidence of cancer following psychological upheavals, but research has also now demonstrated that social stress and loneliness have strong effects on parameters of immune function. Affected particularly are cells termed 'natural killer cells' which are known to play a vital role in preventing the spread of malignant disease. Stressed subjects had significantly lower 'killer cell' activity.[6]

Mentioned above was Lawrence LeShan's observation that loss of relationships or vocations may reactivate earlier difficult childhood emotions and personality problems. It is certainly interesting to speculate whether it is an interaction of underlying personality issues and current stress or trauma, which cause some people to become physically ill after difficult life events whilst others cope. However, he certainly demonstrated the overall connectedness of traumatic life events and cancer in a very elegant predictive study which he performed in 1959.[12] Because of his theory that the loss of a major relationship would predispose an individual to cancer, he predicted that the cancer mortality rate would be highest for widows, next highest for divorcees, next for married people and lowest for those who are single. He analysed data from many earlier epidemiological studies and found that all the data was consistent with his hypothesis.

Muslin looked at 165 women about to have a breast biopsy and found that of those found to have a malignant lump twice as many had just lost a close relationship than those in the benign group.[13] Schmale and Iker also predicted the severity of cervical cancer in a group of women on the basis of life events.[14] However, this area of research is also fraught with enormous difficulty as most of it is retrospective and depends on people's memories of their stresses. It is well known that people's memories of situations and their reactions to them become distorted with time or that they read more into an event when looking back after the occurence of a major trauma. It is almost impossible to provide controls for these sorts of studies too.

To add to the confusion there have been some studies which have failed to demonstrate an association between life events and cancer and some animal experiments which have demonstrated that a chronic social stress producing situation may even be associated with tumour inhibition.[15] Selye in 1979 put forward the theory that some forms of stress may be positively beneficial to the body and it is well observed anecdotally that people get ill when they stop being stressed chronically.[16] This phenomenon is often seen in the 'end of term' colds and 'flus that teachers suffer. It has also been shown that inescapable shock will cause production of tumour in rats more than escapable shock which will produce no such effect and indeed is thought to have a protective effect.[17] What would seem to emerge from these findings is that stress which is in some way controllable by the individual is more beneficial than stress which is uncontrollable, like bereavement. Whilst it is dangerous to extrapolate too much from animal studies, these findings certainly fit with the theory that people who feel less in control in their lives, either due to their basic personalities or their circumstances, have an increased likelihood of getting cancer and a poorer outlook than those who do have a sense of control. It is also interesting in this context to observe that a common definition of a cancer cell is that which describes it as a cell which is out of control.

## Psychological Intervention in Cancer Treatment

The development of these psychological models for susceptibility to cancer has obviously led to the idea that prevention or cure of cancer could occur at the psychological level. The question that then arises is whether or not there is some sort of therapeutic activity which could either:-

1. Return to an individual a sense of control over his or her own destiny in the hope that through some form of communication to the body's cellular level the biological state might be improved,

2. Enable a person's personality to go through a shift whereby their attitudes and coping mechanisms were more consistent with a healthy body,

3. Directly reduce stress levels thereby directly affecting hormonal and immune and nervous functioning, allowing a healthier equilibrium to return.

The techniques which have mainly been employed in an attempt to achieve these objectives have been meditation, imaging or visualisation, relaxation, immune conditioning, hypnosis, spiritual healing and counselling or psychotherapy. For every one of these techniques there are many anecdotal reports of great successes, be they in the form of an increased sense of well-being or at the other extreme, complete remission of disease. Again, although it is extremely difficult to research these sorts of areas, increasing numbers of formal studies are being performed using conventional research tools and it does begin to appear that there is consistency between the various studies.

Both LeShan and Levenson who undertake psychotherapy with cancer patients have many anecdotal reports of the remission of cancer through this technique.[18] A formal study of

'Psychological Intervention in the Treatment of Cancer' performed in 1980 in America reported in summary that "it was found that patients treated with some form of psychotherapy survived twice as long as would have been expected on national averages". It was felt that better patient motivation, greater confidence in treatment and overall positive expectency had contributed to the results.[19]

The Simontons' study of the use of imaging techniques in 1976 showed an average increase in survival time of two times for those using the techniques over those who were not. However some people have found that the original Simonton imagery has only served to increase inner conflict, causing one part of the personality to fight another, hence the use of gentler or more transformative type of imagery described in Chapter 1. Ainslie Meares described a case in his 1978 paper of a patient who achieved a total remission of her advanced cancer using meditation alone, only to suffer a relapse when she started to use aggressive imaging techniques.[20] He postulated that this state of increased alertness or conflict had interfered with the state of mind required for the therapeutic effect of meditation to work. This fits in with ideas in a paper principally on hypnosis written by Lansky in 1982 where he describes a new strategy based on getting patients to "love their tumour to effect self healing".[21]

Hypnosis is often used to help control pain in cancer[21] and to help combat the side effects of treatment but it has also been considered as a treatment in its own right. Bowers commented in 1977 that "if it is true that semantically received information may be somatically coded then the possibility must exist, especially under conditions of deep hypnosis, that some forms of cancer might be helped by hypnotic techniques".[22] Reports from the Newton Centre for Clinical Hypnosis conclude that after eight years of practice it can now be safely said that "not only can hypnosis improve the quality of life, but that it can also prolong it, and indeed that the disease can even be arrested or even reversed by the use of hypnosis alone".

Several reasons have been put forward as to why visualisation and other forms of suggestion may work. One which fits with the above comments is that by focussing the mind on pleasant images and feelings, it can provoke a degree of deep relaxation which reduces stress hormones, thereby allowing the immune system to work more efficiently as the body's autonomic tone shifts from predominantly sympathetic to predominantly parasympathetic. Another idea is that images which bring an accompanying hope and a degree of confidence in one's own will, may have a direct effect on the immune system via the limbic system, mediated through the hypothalamus and pituitary. Dr Meares, who has clear evidence of remission through the use of meditation alone, also postulates that the benefits of meditation are the result of a profound drop in the subjects' anxiety levels with ensuing dramatic changes in hormonal, nervous and immune function.[23] J.R. Cautela has gone as far as describing the concept of immune conditioning, believing that like Pavlov's dogs, human beings could be conditioned by psychological stimuli known to enhance immune functioning.[24]

Spiritual healing must be the hardest of all therapies to research. All reports are anecdotal, such as the witnessed and documented healing of a small boy with Ewing's disease in 1982 at Lourdes.[25] It does seem to appear that some people have a quality of quiet, fearlessness and integration which facilitates others to find the same qualities within themselves, thereby engendering a healthier environment within the body. Of course there may well be quite rational explanations for this phenomenon; for example the influence of the healer may be like force field effects seen in physics when a stronger energy source is placed near to a weaker one. It is certainly true that what a good healer can facilitate in his or her subject at the purely psychological level is that state of being which has so consistently been remarked upon to aid healing: a state of peace.

However there is an inherent dilemma in the use of the therapies discussed above. We have heard from the Greer study that those who fight their cancer do better, but it is a natural outcome of many psychotherapeutic techniques that a patient is brought to a state of acceptance. There exists the paradox of encouraging people to fight while simultaneously trying to reduce their anxiety. One could even argue that achieving a state of acceptance may be contrary to the patients' best interests, as indeed so profound is the state of acceptance in some patients who undergo the transformative experience described in the forthcoming chapters that they really do achieve a state where they become totally accepting of death. However, this type of extremely profound acceptance is usually associated with a great increase in the individual's energy and aliveness and improvement in physical health, and must not be mistaken for the passive acceptance of Greer's group two. The real skill of the counsellor then is to help the patient live that fine line between fighting and acceptance; to enable them to stay in a state of alert and conscious exploration and endeavour.

In his review of *Psychotherapy for Cancer*, Cunningham describes a "pyramid of self healing"[26]. This may help give a guideline to identify those who might be helped by the type of approaches mentioned above. It is a pyramid because he feels that the upper levels have fewer people in them. In order, then, from the bottom of the pyramid, he calls the levels:-

1. Refusal — People who are not aware of their ability to help themselves and are not open to the idea.

2. Possibility — People who are not aware of their ability to help themselves, but are willing to consider the idea.

3. Basic — People who are interested in helping themselves and take basic steps to do so.

4. Follow up — People who learn basic self-help techniques and continue to grow by using them regularly.

5. Advanced — People who pursue self-help at greater depth and increased intensity.

6. Dedicated — People who are dedicated to getting well by self-understanding and control who then help others by sharing their insights.

The first implication from this is that all the techniques described in this chapter will only really be of use to those who are ready or willing to undertake them. The second implication is that they will appeal to probably less than half of the population at any one time. This is really very consistent with what is found in practice. However it must be stressed that even those of category one are sometimes won round by equally stubborn relatives from categories three upwards, only to find they have surprisingly good results! Why these therapies often do not appeal is that they require commitment, work and a degree of faith, because there is no definite promise of cure. However, what makes them attractive is that they do carry hope and a sense of being in control of one's own destiny.

Lerner in his article "Integral Cancer Therapies"[27] describes eight categories of hope. These are:-

1. The realistic hope that one may experience a rare and extraordinary healing (as documented in both the medical and complementary medical literature and in the Bible).

2. The hope that as a patient one belongs to the group who do best for one's particular cancer.

3. The hope of having long disease free intervals.

4. The hope of having sufficient time to reach a desired goal.

5. The hope of being relatively free of psychological and physical suffering.

6. The hope of having minimal side effects from treatment.

7. The hope of having a special time with friends and family and making amends in situations which have previously been intractable.

8. The hope that through illness one may grow in one's being and experience a beauty of life and living, which one might never have achieved before the prospect of dying came so close.

It is with these hopes in mind and an awareness of the evidence pointed to in this article that the Cancer Help Centre staff work with their patients. If as a result of such work a person does have a greater sense of control over their own destiny, and indeed a greater acceptance of him or herself, there need be no further reward for those working in this delicate field.

## Chapter 10

# In their own words ...

## Jim Scott

(*Birth Date*: 4 October 1941)

The surgeon sat on my bed the day after my operation and told me that I had a tumour in my pancreas which he was unable to remove due to the extent of the growth. He said that he had put a bypass into my duodenum so that I could eat (because the tumour was blocking the digestive tract), but that he could not give me radio- or chemotherapy because they had little effect in cases like mine. He was afraid there was no more he could do for me and suggested that "I should put my affairs in order".

Although he had warned me before the operation that this could be the outcome I felt empty, very sad and a little afraid. The more I thought about it, the more I became prepared to die. I am a practising Christian and my faith helped me a great deal. My mother and father had both died of cancer only a few years before and I just felt "Now it's my turn". I have learned since that my reaction was one of a 'passive acceptor'. I suppose I had been like this all my life, accepting whatever happened, seldom arguing or answering back — bottling up my anger, disappointment and sadness. But thank goodness my wife Pat is not like me and said that if there was nothing the doctors could do then we must do something ourselves.

During the time before my operation a friend had given me a book called *A Gentle Way with Cancer*. It contained the 'Bristol Diet' which he thought might help me with my digestive problems. Whilst I lay in hospital Pat read the book and decided this was how we could help ourselves. She came and told me we were going to Bristol. I realised how selfish I was being and that those who loved me could not just accept the seeming inevitability of my death as I was doing. I therefore agreed to go. In the few weeks convalescence before we went to Bristol I read the book myself and became encouraged by some of the case histories in it. The diet seemed to make sense and I began to feel a spark in the part of me that loved a challenge and would let no problem go unsolved.

When I got to the Centre for my stay, I initially found the programme somewhat disturbing, as did several of my fellow residents. We were being asked to expose ourselves; to lay open years of locked up emotions; to ask ouselves questions and face things from the past which we had pushed from our conscious minds, only to have them gnaw away at us from the subconsious. Once I had accepted what I had to do, and with the help of wonderful personal counselling, I began to feel so much more sensitive to life, and to the love I shared with my fellow residents and the staff at the Centre. I also felt a new closeness and awareness in the love I shared with Pat. I still had dreadful feelings of depression but these became fewer as my confidence and belief in my ability to heal myself grew. My mind was getting stronger, despite my weakened body.

I was given spiritual healing for the first time during that visit. Although I felt uncomfortable about having it at first, it turned out to be a powerful experience. Healing is often described as having a cumulative effect, but I think I got 50% of my overall healing in that one session with Christopher Pilkington. Unfortunately, I had to leave the Centre earlier than planned because my stomach was playing up, but I had taken in enough in just over a week to leave with a new strength, and indeed excitement, at the challenge ahead.

Despite my fears that the vegetarian diet would turn me from a once strong fourteen stoner into a bag of skin and bones, I quickly became physically stronger. In fact I felt fitter than I had for years. Pat and I had always had a good marriage but now we seemed to talk and communicate better than ever. The threat to my life has brought us to a oneness which can, perhaps, only be achieved through a crisis like this. Other people began to notice the changes in me next. I was brighter and happier with a new aliveness in my eyes. I had started back to work and here, too, the change was noticed. Though I was as conscientious and keen to work as ever, I didn't allow the job to rule my life, or

allow my workmates to walk over me. They didn't think I was
'as nice a bloke as before' because I stood up for myself if my
judgement was questioned, and if I was annoyed or angry I
showed my feelings. I had learned that my emotions are as much
a part of me as the physical framework which surrounds them
and that they must be shown to be a part of me. I now truly
showed love, joy and sadness and enjoyed the experience
enormously.

Two and a half years since the fight began, I've come down
a little from the high plane I was on for the first year or so. I
am now back to the hurly burly and problems of everyday
living. However, with relaxation and meditation I can cope
with the stress that this creates and if I begin to slip, Pat is
always there to give me a nudge. Physically I am very well. My
surgeon cannot understand it and says that perhaps he made a
mistake in his original diagnosis, but tells me to keep on doing
whatever it is that I am doing.

When I first arrived at the Centre I heard somebody say that
they were glad they'd had cancer. At the time I thought this was
a rash and silly thing to say — but now I think I might agree
with them.

# Helen Kendall
(*Birth Date*: 19 April 1947)

I started suffering with stomach pains and bloating of my
abdomen in 1981. This was diagnosed by my doctor as irritable
bowel syndrome. He felt my condition was probably stress
related. In 1983 another GP offered to do tests but I declined
since I felt I had to find a way of coping with the symptoms and
had decided to try acupuncture. I found my acupuncturist both
sympathetic and optimistic. The treatment was effective in the
short term, relieving my pain, but eventually I began to feel very
unwell again. In 1984 I returned to my GP who sent me for a
barium enema. This revealed that I had a colonic tumour. I was
taken into hospital within three weeks of the diagnosis being
made to have the tumour removed. I was told that I had a
poorly differentiated adenocarcinoma which had infiltrated all
areas of the bowel but had no idea whether my prognosis was
good or not.

My reaction to the diagnosis of cancer was one of complete shock and disbelief. This was not helped by the hospital physician who made very little allowance for my stunned state before rushing on to discuss treatment plans. Part of the reason for the intensity of my reaction was that my mother had died of cancer, and so for me cancer was synonymous with death. It took time for it to sink in, but with the help of friends I slowly began to start thinking about the reality of my situation. Before I went into hospital I made a will and began to talk to my children about the possibility of my dying.

The pain and mental anguish that I suffered whilst in hospital was unbearable. On top of this I had a very bad reaction to some of the drugs that I was given. At one point I felt so ill from them that I thought I was going to die from the treatment. Although the houseman and nurses were pleasant and took good medical care of me, I felt very isolated and frightened. No one in the hospital offered me anything in terms of moral support or counselling. The lack of concern for the quality of life of the elderly, terminally ill patients on the ward also made me very upset. So many of them were ending their lives in a state of anxiety and depression, rather than being allowed to die in dignity and peace. My friends and family enabled me to survive the experience by being with me even when I was unconscious and by constantly giving me their love and support.

I heard about the Cancer Help Centre in 1984 through a friend who had been there and derived great benefit. The first and most important step for me was being helped to fully accept that I had cancer and may die. This really helped me to feel 'normal' again instead of paralysed with fear. Although my friends had been very supportive some found cancer a difficult subject to talk about. At the Centre everyone wanted to talk about it which was an enormous relief and helped me greatly. The counselling, in conjunction with all the other therapies I embarked upon, began to make me feel I had control of my situation and that my prognosis was not totally out of my hands.

The atmosphere of the Centre is deeply healing. Initially I used to visit once a month but now go three monthly. I find it very helpful to see the familiar faces of both staff and patients, and feel both known and loved there. What a contrast to the way I felt in hospital! Paradoxically, my visits to the Centre have helped stop me seeing myself as a 'cancer patient'.

I am convinced now that my cancer was caused partly by stress, rather than by an unhealthy diet (which is thought by more and more scientists to be the likely cause of colonic tumours). At the time that I originally became unwell I was having to cope with the end of a marriage and fears about my future. I was then divorced and moved to a new town where I only knew a few people. The new role of 'single parent' was very demanding; in addition to this I was working full time for the first time since my children were born. I have always been the type of person who has taken responsibility for things that go wrong, even if events were far beyond my control. On top of this, I had never found a way of coping with anxiety that this attitude generated. The counselling that I received at the Centre helped me enormously with this and taught me to accept situations more, rather than struggle with them, and also to look at situations with excitement and insight and to accept the love and support of my family. I learned techniques to diminish my anxiety and the support network of the Centre plus my friends helped me to cope with the practical problems that I had to face. As convinced as I am that my cancer was caused by stress I am equally certain that I have far outlived my prognosis because of the help I have received in learning to deal with it and the strengths that I have since developed.

I would never have imagined it possible that there would be anything to gain from having cancer, but I am genuinely grateful for the opportunity my illness has given me to review my approach to life. I have changed at a fundamental level and I feel happier and more privileged to be alive than before.

# Diana Thompson 'Living with Cancer'

(*Birth Date*: 4 September 1935)

In December 1975, when I had just turned forty, I was diagnosed as having breast cancer. I was immediately given a mastectomy and all was then well until 1981. In that year my health began to deteriorate and by the summer of 1982 I had to go into the Walsgrave Hospital in Coventry, where I had a thorocotomy (operation involving the opening of the chest).

This revealed the presence of multiple secondary cancers in both lungs, the tissue around the heart and in the mediastinal lymph nodes. I was very ill after this operation and the diagnosis was, of course, a shattering blow. When I came home from hospital it took me ten minutes to get up the stairs, being pulled up each step by my husband.

This was the point at which we heard about the Bristol Cancer Help Centre, which had been set up about three years previously to help and encourage people with cancer. It was nearly the end of September before I was able to attend myself, but once I got there I immediately launched into the recommended therapies. At the Centre I experienced a tremendous feeling of peace and hope, and the positive attitude amongst the staff which was wonderfully uplifting — you no longer feel you are struggling on your own. Many are the stories you hear from other patients about how much better they are; even those who several years previously had been given only a few months to live. Obviously, not everyone recovers physically, but even those who do not are considerably helped by the overall care, concern and simply the time that is given to them by the staff, doctors, healers and counsellors. I was encouraged by the Centre staff to continue with my orthodox treatment and took Tamoxifen until July 1986. I slowly gained strength from my new way of life and from the tremendous support I received from my husband, family, friends and the Church.

All seemed to be going well until I had a setback in October 1985. Another secondary was found and removed from my tummy muscle. This temporarily solved the problem, but during the early part of 1986 I began to feel unwell again. In July 1986 it was discovered that the cancer had infiltrated my liver. Not good news. At this point I was taken off Tamoxifen by my consultant, as it did not appear to be holding the cancer any longer. Over the previous few months I had been becoming more and more interested in Iscador treatment and decided to 'give it a whirl'. My doctor, by this time, supported my decision because he felt that Western medicine had no more to offer me. The consultant was also very sympathetic towards my use of Iscador and has in no way written me off because of my decision to try alternatives. I have been on Iscador for a year now and am really feeling very fit on it. My doctor told me recently that when he diagnosed the liver secondaries he thought my life expectancy was about two months. He did not in fact tell me this at the time because I was so enthusiastic about trying the Iscador and he did not want to depress me. Both he and my consultant are quite amazed at how fit I am — long may it remain the case.

Throughout the course of my self-help programme I have set tremendous store by healing. I have a cousin who lives in Liverpool who is a healer; he insists on making the journey to my home weekly to give me healing. I also go to a prayer, meditation and healing group here in Worcester, and a local Cancer Support Group, the maxim of which is that we have to show people that you can live with cancer, not just die with it.

(Diana's story represents the most phenomenal success in self healing terms, as it is now five years since she was found to have her multiple lung secondaries. I am sure that her doctors would have thought that she only had months to live then, let alone when her liver secondaries were diagnosed in 1986!)

# Edna Hill

(*Birth Date*: 6 August 1936)

In 1982 I was diagnosed as having an inoperable brain tumour. I had been completely well up until the day I had a series of fits, which led to the diagnosis being made. The news was therefore a complete shock to me and my husband, Les. In the two months following diagnosis I underwent radio- and chemo-therapy, but still became paralysed down my left side, was unable to read or write and could hardly hear, see or speak. In addition to this I felt extremely ill from the side effects of the treatment.

Les had struggled for the preceding five years with asbestosis, another illness for which there is very little medical treatment. This condition caused him to have such severe breathing problems that he was registered disabled.

He was watching 'Pebble Mill at One' on television one day and saw Rev. Tim Tiley talking about faith healing and the marvellous results being achieved at the Bristol Cancer Help Centre. He was so inspired by this programme that he immediately decided to mount a campaign to overcome our individual illnesses. He brought me to Bristol as soon as was possible. We both went onto a vegan diet and full metabolic supplementation regime straight away, and entered fully into the other aspects of the Centre's programme too. As a result of the diet, counselling and healing both Les and I very quickly felt very much better physically and both enjoyed a great new sense of well-being. To my immense joy, within a few months of starting the Bristol regime, I recovered my full mobility. Within eleven months of my initial collapse I was back at work feeling fit and well and Les was breathing better than he had done for years.

We were so delighted with our results that we felt moved to start a group in Portsmouth where we lived at the time to help other cancer sufferers change their mental attitudes. Since moving to Cornwall in 1984 we have continued this work in our new area. We feel that the hardest battle for the cancer sufferer is to overcome the terrible sense of loneliness and despair that the disease brings in its wake. Our group aims to encourage the members and their families to find a hopeful and positive state of mind by mobilising their spiritual and mental energies. Our approach is based on optimism and example; as we've been through it all, we just want to sit down with a group of people and show them how we've done it.

# Patrick Emsden

(*Birth Date*: 19 November 1919)

I began to suffer with pain and stiffness in my left hip in the Feburary of 1984, seven months after retiring. My GP treated me with anti-inflammatory drugs; understandably she presumed that I had rheumatism. A year later when the pain had got much worse she sent me for X-rays at the Nuffield Orthopaedic Centre (NOC) which revealed the presence of a cyst in the bone. After a biopsy the doctors spoke of 'plasma-cytoma'. The ending 'oma' sounded ominous and I could hardly believe that it was happening to me. My nurse tried to reassure me with, "They can do wonders these days". I left the NOC walking with a stick.

I had fourteen radiotherapy treatments at the Churchill

Hospital during Feburary and March 1985. Things went well
for a few weeks afterwards, then my hip became painful again.
This time X-rays showed crumbling bone. Around that time I
first heard the term 'myeloma' used. Nobody explained it to me
but I understood it to be a form of bone marrow cancer which
seemed pretty serious. The surgeons mentioned the possibility
of an extensive operation to clear the whole area, but to my
relief they decided against this. It became apparent that no
further treatment was planned and that all that was on offer was
built-up footwear to counteract the limp I had developed. The
parting words from the staff at the N.O.C. were "press on".
This made me angry as I felt they were writing me off. By this
time I needed two sticks for walking, a home help, a range of
household aids and was given a disabled sticker for my car.

I was desperate and prepared to try anything. A lay healer in
East Suffolk put me in touch with Hertha Larive, one of the
Centre's highly experienced counsellors and healers, who lived
very close to me. I started seeing her on October 22nd 1985.
Her treatment included discussion, healing, dietary advice,
meditation, imaging and callisthenics. Mrs Larive also loaned
me a number of books which gave me encouragement as well as
food for thought. Talking with her greatly raised my morale.
Her counselling also enabled me to release my anger and
showed me how much energy I was prone to waste on hanging
on to negative emotions. I easily accepted the importance of a
wholesome diet in maintaining a strong immune system.

Around June 1986 I started going to a private physiotherapist
who set me exercises to strengthen my leg. Soon after this I took
up swimming, but gave it up after a while because I was
frightened of slipping over on the wet tiles. I was very cheered
however by the fact that I had proved to myself that I could still
swim. I then bought an exercise bike which has proved
beneficial and safe to use. I also became inspired to go to
Church again for the first time in almost twenty years, but
found so little warmth there that I stopped going regularly. Why
do people look so miserable in Church?

The improvement in my condition after three months of
seeing Mrs Larive was remarkable. I was able to walk with only
one stick again. I no longer needed pain killers and sleeping
pills, and the Bristol Diet ended all my digestive problems. By
July 1986 I had cancelled the home help and returned the

household aids. I am not very good at meditation, but I am quite good at imaging and have a 'helper' — Pallas Athene. I have continued to have quarterly check-ups and my recent X-rays which I have seen show a lot of new bone. The hip joint, which was fuzzy on the first X-rays and very jagged after the crumbling, is now clear cut like a normal joint. Unfortunately, the socket is about an inch higher than normal, accounting for the limp I still have. I believe some of this to be due to the fact that my pelvis is still tilted following the earlier problems, and my next move will be to get the help of a chiropracter to remedy this situation. Even if nothing can be done, I can carry on as I am indefinitely and shall continue the imaging, diet and exercises.

My illness made me realise that my present house and garden in Oxfordshire would be far too big to manage by the time I am much older, and has helped me to decide to move to a much smaller house. I chose to move back to Cambridge because I was so happy there earlier in my life. I moved from Cambridge to Oxford in July 1966, to get promotion and more money. It was about the only decision I have ever made against my better judgement. I also had guilty feelings about interrupting the children's schooling; they were 11, 15, and 17 at the time. But worst of all was my wife's illness, (hepatitis), in April 1967 and her death from cancer of the pancreas in September 1968. The children never settled in Oxford, but have survived and appear none the worse.

I had earlier decided to move back to Cambridge on retirement, but when the time came in 1983 I could not face packing my home into boxes. Although my illness might be considered the last straw, it has given me the energy to undertake a move after all. I know Oxford is not to blame for my experiences, but it will always be associated with a bad period of my life. If I had not been ill, I would probably have spent the rest of my life in Oxford feeling sorry for myself. I now realise that many things I had to part with on moving to the smaller house were not really a part of me, and do not miss them. Above all I feel I am in control of my life. For the first time ever I have learnt to pray. It is not necessary to go to Church, nor even to kneel, but a little thought shows what a lot of things there are to give thanks for. Also, I have realised that there are so many people around us who need our prayers.

In August of this year I made my first plane trip to see my son in Germany. My ambition for next year is not to renew my disabled badge for the car! I am happier now than for many years.

# Barbara Winslade

(*Birth Date*: 23 May 1928)

In the spring and summer of 1985 I began to feel unwell — no pains, but as though I had 'flu and was very run down. I felt tired all the time and had no energy. I then started to get the most excrutiating pain in my right arm. It was not immobilised like a frozen shoulder but ached so much that I could not lie down in bed at night and had to sleep propped up. The doctor gave me pain killers but they did not work at all and after some weeks of this I developed nausea and vomiting. By this time he had taken blood tests but with the development of the sickness he sent me to a consultant.

I was taken straight into hospital for x-rays and tests, thinking in my ignorance that I probably had gall bladder trouble. One of the tests was a liver biopsy. The day after this had been performed, at about lunchtime, in a ward full of women, the consultant walked in with the ward sister and the rest of his team, stood at the foot of my bed and said that he was sorry but I had secondary cancer in my liver and that there was nothing to be done about it. (Where my primary cancer was, no-one knew, but I was told that it would probably manifest itself over the next few weeks). He was pleasant but left me as soon as the news was delivered, leaving me very shocked. The sister was very sweet and kind but had very little to say other than what amounted to 'there there'.

On leaving hospital without knowing what to expect other than an early death, the consultant told me to go and enjoy myself. If I wanted to see him his door was always open and I could go any time (to see him that is!). Luckily, I have a very dear friend who had seen the BBC film on the Bristol Cancer Help Centre. We had a long talk which made me realise that I was very angry at being left 'to get on with it', so I decided to ring Bristol. I was given an appointment two weeks later, and I walked into another world.

The whole concept of the Centre was new to me. The diet was quite a shock, but I embraced it to the letter from the first day. I went to relaxation classes and set about finding a healer locally. I played the tapes I got from the Centre and learnt to 'visualise' and to do 'imaging' to cleanse and heal my body. I was counselled by loving and helpful counsellors and doctors. I had several good crying sessions and learnt to face the problems that I had both ensuing from my illness and from my life in general. I not only learnt how to face my problems but also how to deal with them, and now two years later I know that I have changed. There has also been a terrific improvement in my physical health since following the dietary and supplementation regimes, and having injections of Iscador. I have not felt so well for many years. Mentally, my attitude has improved beyond all recognition. Every day is a bonus and I am conciously thankful for things I had previously taken for granted. Meditation has become very important in my life. I did do a course on meditation, but my healer also teaches meditation and I find his guidance extremely beneficial. I am changing my whole outlook on life and am learning to be more tolerant, loving and helpful to others. People were so good to me when I was ill. I did not know how lucky I was to have so many friends.

My doctor is amazed by my recovery and one day in conversation implied that three months was about my expected life span when I left hospital. I continue to visit the Centre at roughly three monthly intervals, but feel quite a fraud when I am there as I am now so very fit and well. In fact, on my last visit, I used most of my time with the doctor to discuss a minor skin rash! When family commitments allow, I hope to be involved with a local back-up group which is needed so very much in this area.

# Ernest Shepherd

(*Birth Date*: 26 February 1917)

I became ill in late 1980, when, on having a wisdom tooth extracted, I was found to have cancer of the jaw. I then underwent an operation for removal of the left side of my mandible. On waking up from the anaesthetic I was terrified because I discovered that I was unable to talk. I had been warned that learning to speak and eat again would be difficult, but it did not seem as if I could make my mouth work at all. This was not altogether suprising because a day or so later the doctors came back to remove stitches that were holding my tongue in place. No one had explained this to me! In August 1981, just when I was beginning to regain my confidence a lump developed which turned out to be a recurrence in the remaining bone. I therefore underwent an operation to have the lump removed and had an extensive course of radiotherapy. Despite this I had another recurrence in April 1982 in a salivary gland, which was also removed surgically.

Two months later a relative heard about the Cancer Help Centre. I was not sure at first about the relevance of this approach to me, being quite happy to put myself in the hands of my doctors. My first visit to the Centre was therefore more to keep my family happy than from my own initiative. However, on receiving only two or three counselling sessions I realised that although a great deal of wonderful work had been done for me by the surgeons and radiotherapists, I had done nothing for myself; I was always 'stepping back' — this was the missing element. I therefore felt that it was about time that I began to see what I could do and in what way I might be contributing to my illness. I became aware that this pattern of 'stepping back' was very fundamental to my nature and that rather than confronting difficult situations or realising my ambitions, I always tended to be passive, internalising the stress or frustation that this created. My failure to express my feelings had resulted in a life long tendency to depression. In retrospect I became aware that in the period leading up to the emergence of my cancer, due to a number of specific situations I had been taxing this coping mechanism to its limits. It took this illness to make me face my self-destructive way of coping with problems.

It was as if I had suddenly woken up. I gained the courage to attempt two new projects. One of these was a very literal symbol of my desire to rebuild myself. I began to rebuild an old cottage in the grounds of my existing house. The other was that I took up flying again, another symbol of my new found freedom of spirit. Life was suddenly so precious to me. I had been aware that my prognosis was very poor having had a third recurrence, and until coming to the Centre, I had passively accepted this. I can clearly remember the departure of the swallows the first autumn after my visit to the Centre. As I said farewell to them I believed in my heart of hearts that I would never see them again. I did live to see them come back in the Spring of 1983 and 1984, and by this time I was so well that I knew that I would continue to see them for many years to come. In the summer of 1984 I was declared clinically clear, and have now been cancer free for three years.

# Linda Harrison

(*Birth Date*: 24 October 1940)

It was in 1977, when I was 37, that a lump was removed from my left breast and found to be malignant. I had felt quite positive that all would be well as I'd had a lump removed from the same breast a year before which proved benign. Between having the first and second lumps removed my mother died. She had been very ill with emphysema for two years, and had needed constant support and much nursing during this time, so it was, for me, a period of enormous stress and emotion. I was a working actress and was also running a home and looking after my family. It was left to me alone to care for my mother as my sisters were both ill in different ways. One was fighting for her life with bone cancer; the other was in the grip of alcholism. This might give a poor impression of the kind of family I came from. I had an immensely happy childhood with more than my share of love, but none of us were able to cope too well emotionally with the difficulties of life. This, combined with other factors, led us eventually into nothing less than a Greek tragedy!

I see more clearly now how it happened, and am able to understand it with compassion. I was the baby of the family and close to my mother. I loved her dearly, but she too had been an alcoholic, and through her illness and her needs our relationship often became strained. She died in June 1977 and feelings of grief, loss, inadequacy, and most strongly guilt, overwhelmed me for a long period. I didn't know then how it was possible to let go of these emotions, and I clung fast, painful though it was.

Perhaps it was 'the devil I knew'. Worry, anxiety, and the next disaster occurring seemed to be the cross I had to bear. There was no way out.

After my second lump was removed and found to be malignant, I was given a week to prepare for a mastectomy. My prognosis was very bleak because of being young, and after second opinions, which seemed even bleaker, my husband and I felt there was no alternative but to go ahead with it. It was certainly the worst week of our lives, but I filled it as positively as I could by rushing out, buying a freezer, and filling it full of goodies for my husband who would need to do much comfort eating while I was in hospital for three weeks. The news was good after they had operated. They were sure they had removed everything cancerous. Things looked up. I recovered quickly — physically at least. The mental repercussions took a year or so to hit me. I was back at work in an acting, singing and dancing role within a month. I had relied completely on the loving support of my husband and the advice of the doctors. It had all happened so fast that it didn't occur to me then that the cause of my cancer lay, perhaps, deep within me.

The work I was involved in after my mastectomy was very strenuous so it wasn't suprising that another lump came up in my left armpit the following February. After its removal there followed a three week course in radiotherapy, which left me feeling very low. However, my sister with bone cancer had been given only two weeks to live in 1976, and was now a wonderful inspiration to me. As long as she was winning all seemed possible for me. My three monthly check-ups lengthened to six monthly ones, and I was working harder as an actress than ever before. At the five year mark my radiotherapist told me that I was past the danger point and that my cancer was unlikely to return. Life felt safe once more; but during this period I happened to catch a programme on television about the work of the Bristol Cancer Help Centre. It was a revelation to me. This was the way to go about it. Cutting and lopping bits off me wasn't what it was all about at all. Immediately, instinctively, I wanted to go there — to learn that there was something I might do to help myself — to discover the Gentle Way. My body and mind needed kindness above all else. But I was very well, so of course I thought that they wouldn't take me. There were many more people in greater need.

Meanwhile, the family tragedy had continued. My eldest sister died of alcoholism two years after my mother's death and in 1983 my other sister's cancer returned and she died in May of that year. The grief following the loss of my mother and sisters within five years devastated me, and I became less and less able to cope with stress or demands of any kind without crumbling. I was vulnerable in every way. Every infection lowered me that little bit more. I felt incapable of doing my job and this lack of purpose fanned the flames of my worries, anxieties and stresses. Even my marriage which had been happy seemed to be shaky. In November 1984, while I was working on a large leading role in theatre I developed a chest virus which refused to clear up. X-rays revealed shadows on my lungs; a bronchoscopy would be necessary as it was feared the cancer had now spread to my lungs. As it turned out I saved them the trouble of a bronchoscopy, as within three days of hearing this news a lump came up on my diaphragm. Instead they removed this which gave them a one hundred percent certain diagnosis that my cancer had now returned and was probably widespread.

My lovely, sympathetic and now, for the last three years most supportive specialist gave us this sad news and offered me chemotherapy or radiotherapy and the possibility of having my ovaries removed in the hope that this might 'slow things down a bit'. The weekend after I left hospital fate just happened to take us from my home in Leeds to Bristol for a Christmas family reunion. We called in at the Centre, collected the tapes and literature, and felt a good deal calmer after talking to a very lovely nurse. The feel of the place was special to me. It felt like the sort of environment where everything was possible, and therefore, where I would be bound to get well. Many others had done it, so why not me? So, when I got home I went on the diet, and three weeks later I spent a week at the Centre, assimilating the self-help programme of relaxation, meditation, visualisation, diet and healing. I felt daunted but excited by the enormity of the task ahead. At this time, I truly felt I as though I only had a short time to achieve anything. Recently my consultant told me that he had secretly feared that I only had about three months to live at that time. Physically and mentally I was very low. Every time I climbed the stairs I wondered if I would make it to the top. It was into overdrive or nothing! There was, I knew, within me a happy person struggling to unlock her prison bars. All I needed was the help to find that wise soul again — even though it would involve pain.

On returning home I decided to reject the more savage orthodox treatments of chemo- and radiotherapy, although I did accept Tamoxifen. The quality of life was of vital importance to me, not the quantity. I have been taking Tamoxifen for three years now and have had no side effects from it at all. However, even before I started to take it the X-rays had shown a regression of the tumour in my lungs and my friends had all commented on how much better I was looking since starting the Bristol regime. The first thing that people noticed was how much clearer my skin and eyes were, and this really helped prove to me that the diet was working. The diet also helped my diabetes. I had been diabetic from the age of fifteen so it was no joke having to accept yet another diet. But now I found I could give myself less insulin, eat more carbohydrates, and suffer fewer hypoglycaemic attacks. I also enjoyed the food and despite the hard work I've changed from being a creative French cook into a creative raw energy one. The other therapies, relaxation, meditation and counselling were new to me, but my sister and I had discovered a marvellous healer, the famous E.G. Fricker, when she had been ill. I travelled to London to see him whenever I could.

During the next year I continued to improve remarkably. My cancer cells were regressing. I continued to follow the self-help programme (which took discipline), but was only well enough to do the odd radio play. What mattered most was getting well again.

I found, through working with my remarkable Bristolian Counsellor, Barbara Siddall, that it was possible to free myself of habit patterns I had been locked in for years. I found myself re-discovering joy in life. One major example happened one freezing cold day. Cancer cells don't like oxygen, so I walked as much as possible. I found, because the wind was so cold and strong that at one point I couldn't go either forwards or backwards, the wind had taken what little breath I had away. So I asked the trees for help and in a short time I was able to walk a small distance, gradually becoming able to walk further as the energy from the trees revived me. Eventually, I discovered that I had been walking for at least an hour. This led me more and more, in all sorts of subtle but tangible ways to tap into the healing power of nature. It can reach and give us so much if we open up to it. I had forgotten it existed, and re-discovered it by chance.

Initially, after returning from my first visit to Bristol, I had a difficult few weeks setting things in motion. Leeds, I was informed, was something of a desert where alternative therapies were concerned. Although this was frustrating to begin with, quite the reverse proved to be true. I found a counsellor not too far away; Dr Arthur Bailey, a remarkable teacher to whom I owe so much and to whom I will be forever grateful. I met and talked with many others, including cancer sufferers who had recovered in their own remarkable ways. I tried Cranial Osteo-pathy and Homoeopathy in an attempt to stimulate my immune system. I found both very beneficial. I also attempted other positive therapies such as reflexology, iridology and autogenic training. The latter aided me to obtain a deeply relaxed state in meditation. Nearly all of these I found in or around Leeds. I also gave myself occasional courses of Iscador injections.

Most of all I had to learn, and it's still an on-going process, how to let go of the vast amount of guilt, pain, anger, fear and resentment that had built up. This proved to be painful but also helped me to rediscover my own creativity, which was an uplifting and profoundly liberating experience. It was a pure and tangible healing process, leading me towards an inner freedom I had never thought possible, and which I'm still excited by. Of course there have been many bad times when fear and doubt crept in; many times when I thought I wouldn't make it. Our conditioning gives us so many hang-ups about losing. It's three years since I was given three months to live, and even now it's not always easy to put trust in myself, to continue showing myself kindness and encouragement. Lumps appear from time to time. Fear clamours for attention again, together with worry and anxiety, such old and well established habit patterns with me. This powerful trio fills, all too easily, the gaps just filled with newly established peace. The answers in my meditations continue to be simple. Encourage the peace and let the fear fall away.

Seneca, the philosopher, as long ago as 4 BC, knew what it was all about when he said, "Remember before all else, to strip things of all that disturbs and confuses you, and to see what each is at the bottom; you will then comprehend that they contain nothing to fear except fear itself." It's taking time for me to assimilate this most wise advice, but slowly the light is dawning. For me it was not as for some 'a blinding light on the road to Damascus'. However, I am now back working full time, both in theatre and radio. I am using my experience of the last three years and hope to do more in the way of counselling and healing. There is so much I have been given that I can share with others.

I feel extremely lucky, because my specialist has been both supportive and approving of the help I've received from Bristol. He can see how well I am and I now feel views me holistically. He has been content to monitor rather than excise a lump that appeared recently. The lump is, at this moment, getting smaller and I believe it will go; if it doesn't the prospect of living with a lump doesn't alarm me as it used to do. I have lived with lumps and bumps for years that haven't been removed or proved to be cancerous. I am paying attention to this lump, but I'm not giving it any encouragement! It's only the size of a pea and at the moment I'm in the process of deciphering its code message to me. I know that I'm more in control than ever before. I don't look like a person who is about to die. As someone who hadn't seen me for years said, "You look far more robust".

I've never been afraid of dying, only the process of how it might happen. It's natural and easy to fear the prospect of dying of cancer. We've been conditioned into the fear of it for years. What we need so much to do is to learn to treat it as any other disease; something we can recover from. The root of our problems stems from the medical profession's fear of cancer; something that is incurable. I completely agree with Penny Brohn when she says that we need to create a new reality for ourselves; one that requires us to be alive. It is up to us to pass this message on whenever we can. Also to accept that, however small, we are part of the wondrous evolution of the universe, capable of finding the joy of life in every moment.

The word 'prognosis' means nothing to me now. It has become meaningless, which shows me clearly that fear clouds one's ability to see the truth. When death finally comes, I hope that if fear is around I shall be able to let it go. I hope that with the gifts I've been given over the last three years, I shall be fully open to experience its presence and the awe-inspiring challenge of change that it will bring me. It is, after all, what life is preparing us for. Not one of us knows, until it happens, what it will be like. I hope, as Peter Pan says, "It will be an awfully big adventure", but at the moment I'm far too busy with life!

## Chapter 11

# The Summary

It will be easy for any doctors or scientists reading this book to dismiss these cases as no different medically from the small percentage of patients who have unexpected remissions of their illnesses while undergoing conventional treatment. All consultants have a handful of patients who have proved all prognostications wrong without having consciously 'taken the situation into their own hands' in any way. They might easily say that to pick out these 'successes' and postulate that one is seeing a distinct phenomenon, without having any statistical data to back up this assertion, is completely absurd. However, despite having no statistics whatsoever to prove it, I am convinced that I have seen results which point to the existence of tangible connections between the nervous, endocrine and immune systems and all the tissues of the body; in other words, the body and mind. This is why I have decided to stick my neck out and write up these cases. As far as I am concerned all science begins with intuition, observation and anecdotal reporting. Rationalisation and quantification follows. I would therefore encourage the scientific community to ponder this phenomenon seriously, as the implications are enormous.

It must be said that on the basis of the overall statistics which are emerging at the Cancer Help Centre, the number of people who embark upon a self-healing programme for the treatment of cancer who achieve complete remission is small. (But it is most important to see this in the context of the society in which we live which has an all-pervasive medical model which gives us the 'knowledge' that this is not possible.) It does however appear that many achieve an extension in their medical 'life-expectancy', and almost all experience an improvement in their physical and mental states. There are many people though, for whom the approach is completely nonsensical, who, either with or without having really inspected it, feel unable to take it on. This is usually because of their complete commitment to 'science' or the medical model, or because at the bottom line their real commitment to staying alive is weak or non-existent. It may also be that they find the initial discomfort that can be entailed in this process too much to cope with in addition to the burden of the disease itself. Yet another reason is that others like or feel very secure in their present self-image or personality, and feel that to allow the possibility of a personality shift, or change in attitudes, life-style or behaviour would be to betray or lose themselves.

It must be clearly stressed again that the Centre does not present itself as a treatment centre, or in any way imply that its goal is the cure of cancer. In choosing a set of cases to write up which illustrate the very best outcomes of the Centre's approach, I do not intend to imply that all cancer is curable through this approach or to give a distorted boost to the Centre's public image. What I do intend is that in the process of describing this inspiring humanitarian project I will help to reawaken the medical profession to the interconnectedness of mind, body and spirit which these cases illustrate so well. I hope by doing this that more doctors and scientists will become inspired to research and use this phenomenon both to increase our understanding and to assist in the eternal battle to lessen human suffering.

# The Phenomenon

When in her hospital bed, faced with the diagnosis of cancer and the offer of a mastectomy Penny Brohn knew that there was another way round this problem.

I have always felt that the state of a person's energy had far reaching consequences, both on their own health and the health of those around them. I knew that in an instant, the entrance into the room of someone who was bright, happy, inspired or dynamic could change the subjective reality of everyone around them. Each person's perception of their world, internal and external, could change in seconds. Physical aches and pains could disappear, and what before had been perceived as a problem causing the creation of mountains of mental resistance could more or less evaporate. I also observed the way that a child's tummy ache could disappear in seconds upon the announcement of an exciting outing, or that an old person could die within six weeks of losing their spouse. I was left in no doubt whatsoever of the connection between a person's emotional state, mental state, overall energy and the state of their physical health. Penny and Pat, Christopher and Alec created a place where these intuitions could be tested and as predicted, medical expectation has repeatedly been stood on its head.

Many doctors and scientists are prepared to acknowledge that changing one's perception of a problem can greatly diminish the suffering involved, but few are prepared to acknowledge that changing one's perception of a situation can alter the material reality. We have the gate theory of the perception of pain[1] which acknowledges that pain perception is a very changeable phenomenon depending on the other nervous input to the pain circuits. One could argue that by filling the mind of a suffering individual with all sorts of positive thoughts and distractions one is purely diminishing the time spent feeling anxiety and fear. It could also be said that what is achieved at Bristol is that individuals are brought into a state of acceptance of their fate by repeatedly discussing their situation. I am sure that these two phenomena do occur, but am now quite convinced that it goes further and that what have previously been thought of as 'unchangeable bodily functions' as well as disease processes, can be changed by one's state of mind and energy level.

It has therefore been immensely gratifying to come across such stunning examples of this phenomenon in such cases as those I have presented from the Bristol Cancer Help Centre. These are just a few hand-picked examples which represent hundreds of patients who have arrived at Bristol in the most depleted of physical states, and have seen their physical symptoms drop away as their energy levels and state of mind have been steadily improved with intense encouragement, love and support and nourishment of all aspects of their beings. Through juggling with their realities and truths, the rigid belief system which keeps them trapped in the notion that they are going to die is eroded and replaced with a belief in themselves, their own power, and their ability to take control of their own life and decisions. It would appear that as their inner beliefs and expectations change, so their outer reality follows suit, mirroring exactly these new beliefs.

Quite often fear itself is the energising factor, especially once the mental barrier to perceiving the true danger and threat to life has been dropped. In this respect death itself can be seen as the greatest teacher; its approach throwing all that is possible in life into sharp relief. In other cases it is the joy of unconditional acceptance, or the liberation of experiencing ego-free states of consciousness, or for yet others the sheer excitement of being given permission to express themselves which provides the fuel which brings them back to life. The skill of the therapists then, is to endeavour to find what is keeping the energy trapped and help liberate it while providing enormous support to allow the person to feel safe enough to do this. The whole process is rather like rekindling the glowing embers of a dying fire, gently feeding it and bringing it back into life. It may take time and patience at first to get the flames going, and care must be taken not to put it out in the process but once the fire is alight it is easy to stoke it up into a brilliant blaze.

When I had a psychiatry post I was fascinated to observe the reverse phenomenon. I saw mental states change radically when changes occured at the physical level. For example two chronic schizophrenics became moderately 'normal' mentally as they developed physical illnesses. One old lady's delusions would wax and wane with the remission and exacerbation of her Chrohn's disease and another very anarchic, loud and aggressive lady became completely 'tame' as she developed a cancer of the rectum. I am not extrapolating that the state of mind created by the Bristol approach is schizophrenic; the similarity is that the cancer patient arrives in a mentally and energetically 'contracted' state and proceeds to open up, in so doing losing physical symptoms. The schizophrenic is in a very open, energised mental state which 'contracts' as the cancer or physical illness develops, with the loss of mental symptoms.

Dr Richard Moss[2] takes this notion of expanded and contracted states further using it to describe situations as well as individual states. For example he would say that the reason I felt the individuality draining out of me when I walked into a hospital environment was because it was an energetically contracted environment and I was having to shrink to fit. He would say that a bright dynamic alive person is energetically expanded and that if their energy is consistent, they will create the 'space' for everyone around them to 'expand'. If their energy is a little more shaky then they themselves will contract to take on the 'energy' of their surroundings. Maybe when people express their feeling of relief on walking through the doors of the Cancer Help Centre what they are describing is the relief of entering an energetically expansive place. The mantle that has been thrust upon them by the diagnosis and fear of death feels constricting and uncomfortable as do the restrictions placed upon them by their conditioning and circumstances. In energetic terms they are suddenly able to expand out of these rigid energetic structures and breathe again, because fear loses its power in the presence of so much love.

Why the Centre feels this way is open to speculation. We are used to places full of sick people being hushed, sad and depressing. Many have described the atmosphere at the Centre as one of quiet and determined optimism. The non-judgemental expansive atmosphere creates for many the nearest to a sense of home-coming that they can ever remember experiencing. It may feel this way because of the individual states and attitudes of those running the Centre. Most of the people in the Centre practise what they preach and many of them have beliefs and philosophies which allow them to have no fear of death themselves. All acknowledge that anything is possible. Most of the staff are acutely sensitive to their effect on everyone else, and take pains to shed distorting burdens by seeking help from each other, through being counselled or belonging to support groups.

The result is that the atmosphere is very alive. Not in any frantic sense, but with a feeling of growth and renaissance. The other factor to be considered is the psychic and spiritual input to the Centre. There are many people, but in particular Canon Christopher Pilkington, who spend hours every day praying for and meditating upon the Centre, in order to set up and maintain a healing atmosphere. In the past, too, the Centre was a convent, which is believed by some to have left its imprint on the atmosphere of the building (although the early Centre at Downfield Road was an ordinary house and many people reported just as strong a sense of relief on entering that building). The other vital factor is that so much love and positive intention is generated in the course of a day's work at the Centre and there is such a sense of fellowship and combined

purpose. One could argue that a huge amount of tension, anger
and fear is also expressed within the Centre, but the net effect
is that the atmosphere contains a wonderful combination of
aliveness, peacefulness and love.

Lawrence LeShan[3] also feels that the central key to Holistic
medicine is the process of enlivenment and thus raising of the
energy level of the individual. He will spend hours helping his
clients to discover or remember an area of life which really
excites and fulfills them, however contrary that might be to
their conditioning, pressures or current lifestyle. He will follow
any cue that an individual can remember of a time, event or
circumstance which made them feel really enthusiastic and alive
and encourage the person to recreate these situations or
pastimes in ways appropriate to their present circumstances.
This often results in people making radical changes in their
lifestyle or occupation; often with tremendous improvements in
their physical health ensuing. He calls this helping a person to
"sing their own song" and says that you know when this is
happening because, like a child on Christmas eve, you are so
excited that you can hardly bear to go to sleep, because you are
so keen for the next day to come. This is just what many of the
patients report having shed their enormous burdens; that there
is so much catching up on 'living' to do that each day seems just
too short.

The creation of the contracted, sad, disabled and depressed
state in which many people exist occurs, I believe, because of a
combination of personal suffering and repeated emotional
defeats in conjunction with prevailing belief systems, political
systems, social conditioning — combined overall expectations
which dictate how a person should behave and what they are
capable of. It is my belief that in the very heightened state
brought about by the fear of death or the loss of personal
security that an individual can discover that they have more
power and knowledge than they could have ever imagined
possible.

A wonderful example of this is the true story of *The
Marvellous Adventure of Carbeza de Vaca* by Haniel Long.[4]
This is the story of Nunez Carbeza de Vaca, a Spanish con-
quistador who was shipwrecked on the Isthmus of Panama.
Along with a handful of survivors, he made an extremely
dangerous journey, often as the prisoner of native Indians,

across the isthmus in the search for other Spaniards and his possible return home. They themselves became extremely ill but were also surrounded by unspeakable poverty and suffering within the Indian communities with which they travelled. Haniel Long describes this as the tale of "what man can do when he must do something or die". The Indians, believing these bizarre people who had come from the sea to have magical powers, commanded them to heal the sick of their communities. If they could not do this they would be killed as they could not possibly feed the extra mouths of their prisoners if they were of no special value.

In the terror, bewilderment and complete disorientation of their situation they prayed and prayed and prayed to be given the power of healing and to their utter amazement, the Indians brought before them became healed. Once their healing abilities had been demonstrated, Indians were brought to them in droves for healing, with success time and time again. Nunez writes, "In the effort of praying I have felt as though something in me had broken to give me the power of healing. Alone in this wilderness no tissue of the body hindered the mysterious power." He goes on to say that "being Europeans, we thought that we had given away to doctors and priests our ability to heal. But here it was, still in our possession. We were more than we thought we were." "Those eyes . . ." he exclaims, "they thrust me out of myself into a world where nothing, if done for another, is impossible".

At the end of his tale, which is his report to King Charles, he describes how he does finally discover a community of Spaniards, but far from being relieved, he finds himself utterly horrified and disgusted to meet "the men he used to be". He cannot bear to see the arrogance, insensitivity and ignorance of his fellow Spaniards. Initially, he extends his healing abilities to his compatriots, but as he becomes reintegrated into his community his powers fade as he becomes 'safe' again. He concludes by saying that "our communal life dries up our milk. We regard our native land as a power which acts of itself and relieves us each of exertion where plenty abounds. We surrender our generosity believing our country replaces us each and several. This is not so and is indeed a delusion. On the contrary the power of maintaining life in others lives within each of us, and from each of us does recede if unused."

Many patients with cancer are in a similar position to Nunez; they must do something or die. However, they are surrounded by the belief that there is nothing that they can do to help themselves and often the person who is saying this most forcefully is the doctor to whom they have 'given' all the power. The reaction of most is to succumb to this reality as it is so heavily endorsed by the society and people surrounding them. However, it is now quite clear from the Centre's experience that others faced with this existential crisis, can, like those sailors, discover extraordinary hidden potential in themselves and their environment. This idea of the limiting of our potential by our expectations and beliefs fits entirely with Illich's notion of a 'Deschooling Society'[5] which, in the imposing of external control, security and education, robs individuals of their own power and knowledge.

## The Researchability of the Approach

Any approach to illness which has made claims of cure or complete remission of disease is subject to a barrage of demands for proof. Proof in the 1980's means statistical evidence, and to be really valid that must be as a result of randomised, double blind prospective trials. What randomised means is that all subjects being studied must be allocated at random to the different study groups A, B, and C (i.e. the group receiving treatment A, the group receiving treatment B, and a control group C receiving no treatment). What double blind means is that neither the subjects nor the people who are judging the effects of the treatment, or lack of it, know which group the subject is in. Prospective means that data cannot be collected from the past as this too may distort the facts, so the study must use completely new material and will therefore take many years from the setting up of the trial to yield results. The other prerequisite is that subjects studied are 'matched' as nearly as possible for as many factors as possible, e.g. age, sex, social status, staging and type of disease, etc, etc. One can see at a glance that this set of requirements is almost completely impossible for an approach such as that used at Bristol.

To start, with people cannot be allocated randomly to different treatment groups in this instance, since almost everyone has very strong views about whether they wish to pursue Bristol type treatment or purely conventional treatment. It is impossible that subjects would not know which study group they are in, and the normal idea of matching becomes impossible when subtle psychological characteristics in combination with particular life events are thought to be important variables. This means that conventional research becomes almost completely impossible in all but the crudest of terms. Many doctors share Dr Cullen's view that the results from Bristol are very biased even now, because it is a self-selected group of highly motivated individuals who come to the Centre. I would certainly agree that the results are related to the type and motivation of the people who come, because I believe entirely that it is patients' attitudes which change the outcome of their illness, and not the therapy per se. I'm sure this variable, as well as the placebo effect and the effects of charismatic and optimistic doctors, also affect the success of the approach, but I know that this is also the case in orthodox medical settings. These factors are, however, rarely taken into account in the evaluation of conventional treatment.

Despite feeling so strongly about motivation being a crucial factor, I must add that a small subset of the people, like Ernest Shepherd, come to Bristol because they 'feel they should' for their relatives' sake and so are not genuinely motivated initially. Many are quite sceptical about all, or certainly parts, of the therapy, but it is astounding how many of these people become committed to their self-help practices once they begin to feel positive effects. Many who started out feeling completely at the mercy of their illness have found the real motivation several months into their programme, like Mary and Jim. It would therefore seem that the effects are not entirely dependent on initial motivation.

Another difficulty of researching many branches of alternative medicine, as highlighted by the Research Council for Complementary Medicine (RCCM) in their annual conferences on the subject,[6] is the inseparability of the effects of the treatment per se and the effect of the individual therapist. A further complication at Bristol is the multifactorial nature of the approach, and of course there is the problem described by Heisenburg in his 'Uncertainty Principle' that the very act of observation of a process changes it. The RCCM are presently wrestling with these problems because, until there is any 'hard scientific evidence', the medical profession can all too easily dismiss the alternatives, or worse still can outlaw them, as has happened in many other countries of the world.

For all of the reasons mentioned above I think it will be nigh on impossible to get the kind of data that the medical profession is used to out of the Bristol Cancer Help Centre. I feel that what is far more likely is that in the next decade the budding subject of psycho-neuro-immunology will continue to tie up the connections between the immune, hormonal and nervous systems, demonstrating the effects of differing moods and mental states on all aspects of human physiology. This phenomenon is particularly well illustrated by the recently described 'failure to thrive syndrome' where it has been shown that despite adequate metabolic nutrition, in the absence of adequate emotional provision a child will fail to grow physically.

Proof of this interconnectedness will force doctors and politicians to acknowledge just how basic the connections are between a person's mental and physical states, which in turn will demonstrate how vital it is to take into account the mental states created by educational, family and work environments, and religious, political and social systems. It will be seen to be necessary to take mental state into account in the designing of any preventative medical programmes and the physical risk to individuals coping with very difficult life events will finally be appreciated. This could even allow for the development of facilities to enable the giving of special care and nurturing for those who are suffering severe loss and stress, in order to help prevent the ever-continuing cycle of grief and illness causing more illness and grief. This is certainly the next priority on the programme of the Bristol Cancer Help Centre, along with research into the development of Holistic Medical Education, both for those entering the caring professions and for all school children.

# The Transferability of the Approach to the N.H.S.

One of the obvious limitations of the Centre's approach is the relatively small number of people that it can serve and the fact that visiting the Centre costs money. As stated previously, the development around the country of local cancer support groups makes the approach ever more available. Also, the existence of a bursary fund means that no one is turned away from the Centre on financial grounds. However, the numbers who benefit directly are obviously small, and while it is viewed as a fringe approach there will be bound to be scepticism by the public and the medical profession. No one who practises at Bristol is happy about the fact that patients have to pay four-fifths of the cost of their treatment (the rest coming from charitable donation), but as yet strenuous attempts to have it N.H.S. funded have failed. The next obvious question, then, is that if this approach is found or believed to be valid, could it not be transferred into the present N.H.S. system and hence become available to all routinely, and indeed, if it was available to all routinely, would it still work?

As I have mentioned earlier, I feel that part of the phenomenon occurs precisely because people come to the realisation that they have to find out how to get themselves better. Like the sailors on the Isthmus, they find their power when they only have themselves to rely on. This is analogous to alcoholic 'rock-bottom'. Because the present medical assumption is that all power, knowledge and ability to make changes lies with the medical professionals, and that there really is nothing that a person can do to affect the outcome of their own illness, it would appear to be nigh on impossible for people to activate their self-healing potential within the present medical context. It is well understood by pyschiatrists that alcoholics must find their true commitment to life before recovery can occur. As yet this concept has not entered the realms of physical medicine.

Before this can be achieved, the most basic beliefs of the medical profession will have to shift or broaden, so that it is understood that in many cases it is not controlling an individual which makes him healthy, but supporting him so that he can learn to look after himself. This is why it is so urgent for the psycho-neuro-immunologists to prove the interconnectedness of mental state and physical state. The state of loss of control, and the apathy and depression it brings with it, are, I believe amongst the most damaging states of mind to the health of the individual. The present medical belief system not only fails to encourage individuals to work on finding their health but actually disables them by telling them that there is nothing they can do.

One must also consider the question of the kind of time and attention which people receive. The scientific model has led to the practice of delivering cold, clinical care. In surveys carried out over the last decade people have repeatedly said, to the amazement of the profession, that they rate the personality and warmth of their doctor above his or her knowledge and skill. I believe that a vital part of the recovery process is dependent upon the quality of the relationship between the doctors/nurses and patients, which in turn depends upon the quality of their relationship with themselves and their own mental states. I am sure that there is a natural reciprocity between the needs of doctors, nurses and their patients which has been obscured by the intellectualisation of medicine. Patients desire to be cared for and doctors and nurses desire to care for them, but modern medical priorities demand that we do otherwise.

In our frantic attempts to assess, quantify and treat symptoms we often fail to greet, contact or comfort the patient at all. The treatments often make people feel worse rather than better, and worse still, sometimes do greater and more lasting damage than was likely to be caused by the disease itself. In the process the doctors and nurses become exhausted and disillusioned, and are no longer in a position to inspire hope and confidence themselves. The absence of any real concern by the profession for the individual states of its staff is well illustrated by junior medical staffing policies. Junior doctors work absolutely ridiculous hours at present. In one job I had in 1983 I was required to work 88 hours and 136 hours on alternate weeks for six months! (There are only 168 hours in the week.)

It is common knowledge that we can't help other people emotionally if we are exhausted and stressed ourselves. I have been in such a state myself after a 36 hour shift that I have had to be looked after by the patients, who seemed to be the only people who realised that all was not well! I remember sobbing in the arms of a poor alarmed patient in the Ladies of the x-ray department, after one such stint when my bleep had just gone off for the fifth time in ten minutes, the staff of the x-ray department would not co-operate and arrange the tests my consultant was insisting I should get done that day, and I knew I had about ten more jobs to do before I could go home.

I am not alone in feeling this way. Any junior doctor can recall such moments. One young doctor told me that on coming into the hospital to do a weekend obstetric shift he felt not only as if he was coming into prison, but worse still, as if he was going into solitary confinement. He knew perfectly well that there would not even be a five minute break from 9 o'clock on Friday morning until 5 o'clock on Monday evening when he could fully relax. He would get very little sleep, and what sleep he did get would be interrupted at one or two hourly intervals. He knew that there would be no-one around for him to talk to or get support, encouragement or praise from. The nurses and patients would expect and hope that he be bright, willing, enthusiastic and in control, and would be understandably upset if he were not, when at heart he would be feeling tired, lonely, depressed and rather frightened by his responsibility. People sometimes argue that for doctors to complain about their working conditions is contrary to the spirit of service, but I believe that unless they are aware of and can look after their own needs they will never understand or value the needs of others, or worse, never be able to help others do the same, thereby keeping them ever dependent on a paternalistic medical system.

Of course, I do agree with some of the patients quoted in this book that there are some aspects of the Centre's approach which could be transferred into the existing system; for example, attention could be given to diet and its supplementation, and counselling and healing could occur as long as outside, rested people could be brought in to do it! Indeed, some oncology departments have already begun to offer a counselling service to their patients. However, I am concerned that the type of counselling offered, by and large, may just be of the 'there there' variety, designed to get people to accept the medical reality of the situation rather than to explain and discuss the possible choices, (including not having any treatment at all). The former type of counselling would be better than none, allowing the expression of feelings and fears, but would certainly not allow for the exploration of the creative or transformative possibilities of the situation.

In summary then, I would have to say that while I applaud individual efforts to take holism into the N.H.S. setting, I feel that there needs to be a complete revolution in medical thinking, training and practice before patients can receive anything like the feeling of unconditional love, relief and autonomy that they get from the Bristol Cancer Help Centre. It is this unconditional support which is vital to enable people to confront their most difficult issues, which is in turn necessary if they are to find a state of mental, and therefore physical, equilibrium. I also recognise the power for many of a period 'in the wilderness' without support during which they can have vital insights, rediscover their priorities and choose life rather than death. They can then truly embark upon the pilgrimage to find their health. The path is still hard once they have reached this decision, but almost impossible before. I therefore feel that the fact that the holistic approach has to be sought out at present is true to its essence and may well be part of its success, and that the starkness of the medical reality is often a completely integral part of the resurrection process. Indeed, Penny herself has said that if people had been even a little gentler and more patient with her right at the beginning when she had her first biopsy, she would probably have been persuaded to have the mastectomy and there may well have been no Bristol Cancer Help Centre at all!

There is a great deal of food for thought contained within these pages for all health care professionals, but the most fundamental and recurrent plea of all the patients at the Centre which can be absorbed and practiced by any doctor, is that they never tell a patient when they are going to die. As Penny says, this immediately risks becoming a self-fulfilling prophecy. On the other hand, nearly all agree that there is a need to know that their life is truly threatened, because otherwise they are not given the chance to fight for it. The final message, every bit as important as the foregoing two, is that doctors should constantly bear in mind that they do not know the whole answer, and should therefore never take it upon themselves to be the final arbiters of what is and is not possible. They must resist giving announcements of the final and complete truth. As Veronica Mills so beautifully puts it: "If they close one door, they must open another".

# References

## Chapter 1

1 Brohn, Penny: *Gentle Giants*. Century.
   *The Bristol Programme*. Century.

2 "Changing 'Unchangeable' Bodily Processes by Hypnotic Suggestions".
   *Advances* (Jour.Inst.Advancement of Health) Vol 1, Number 2: Spring
   1984.

3 a. Gerson, Max: *The Gerson Therapy*.
   b. Passwater, Richard: *Cancer and its Nutritional Therapies*. Pivot
   Books.

4 Rippon, Saddhya: *The Bristol Recipe Book*. Century.

5 Patel, Dr Chandra: *Fighting Heart Disease*. Dorling and Kindersley.

6 Lysbeth, Andre von: *Pranayama*.

7 a. Pauling & Cameron: *Cancer and Vitamin C*. The Linus Pauling
   Inst. of Science and Medicine.1979. (Review of Megavitamin
   Therapy)
   b. Cameron, Pauling & Leibovitz: "Ascorbic Acid and Cancer: A
   Review", *Cancer Research* 39, 663-681 March 1979.

8 Wald et al: "Plasma Retinol, Beta Carotene and Vitamin E levels in
   relation to the future risk of breast cancer." *Brit.Jour.Cancer* 1984,
   49, 321–324.

9 a. Salonen et al: "Selenium, Vitamin A and E serum levels correlated
   with the future cancer deaths." *Brit.Med.Jour.* Feb 9th, 1978.
   b. Young, V.R.: "Selenium, a case for its essentiality in man." *New
   Eng. Jour. Med.* May 14 1981.
   c. "Selenium perspective." *Lancet.* March 26, 1983.

10 *Iscador: Use of and research references:* Weleda Ltd, Heanor Rd,
   Ilkeston, Derbyshire.

11 Centre for Transpersonal Psychology, 7 Pembridge Place, Notting Hill
   Gate, London, W.11.

12 Fifield, Lionel & Burling, Joy: Tapes and Affirmation Cards. c/o
   Cancer Help Centre, Bristol.

13 Meditation Techniques as taught by the Friends of the Western
   Buddhist Order: books and courses from 9 Cromwell Rd, St.
   Andrews, Bristol.

14 Simonton, O.C.: *Getting Well Again*. Bantam.

15 LeShan, Lawrence: *How to Meditate*. Thorsons.
   Meares, Dr Ainslie: *The Wealth Within*. Ashgrove.

16  Young, Alan: *Spiritual Healing, Miracle or Mirage.* DeVorss (USA).
    Herzberg, Eileen: *Spiritual Healing: A Patient's Guide.* Thorsons.


## Chapter 9


1   Evans, E.: *A Psychological Study of Cancer.* Dodd, Mead (USA)
    (1926).

2   Kissen, D.M.: "The Significance of personality in lung cancer in men."
    Annals of N.Y. Acad. Sci. 125, 820–826 (1926).

3   Schmale, A.H. & Iker, H.D. "Hopelessness as a predictor of cervical
    cancer". Soc. Sci. Med. no.5, 95–100 (1971).

4   Thomas, C.F. & Duszynski, K.R. "Closeness to parents and the
    family constellation in a prospective study of five disease states;
    suicide, mental illness, malignant tumour, hypertension and and
    coronary heart disease." *Johns Hopkins Med.Jour.* 134, 251-270
    (1974).

5   Pettingale, K.W., Greer S. and Dudley, E.H.T.: "Serum IgA and
    emotional expression in breast cancer patients." *Jour.Psychosom.Res.*
    21, 395–399 (1977).

6   LeShan, L.L.: *You Can Fight for your Life.* Evans (USA).

7   Greer, S. Morris, T. & Pettingale, K.W.: "Psychological response to
    breast cancer: effect on outcome". *Lancet* 2, 785–787.

8   Stavray, K.M., Buck, O.W., Lott, S.S & Wanklin, J.M.: "Psycho-
    logical factors in the outcome of human cancer." *Jour.Psychsom.Res.*
    12, 251–259

9   Temoshok, L. "Personality, coping style, emotion and cancer: towards
    and integrative model." *Cancer Surveys* Vol 6, no 3, 545–565 (1987).

10  Derogatis, L.R., Abeloff, M.D. and Melisaratos, N.: "Psychological
    coping mechanisms and survival time in metastatic breast cancer."
    *Jour.Alt.Med.Asn.* 242, 1504–1508 (1979).

11  Kay, N.E. & Morley, J.E.: American Federation for Clinical Research
    Meeting (1983).

12  Muslin, H.L., Gyarfas, K. & Pieper, W.J.: "Separation experience and
    cancer of the breast." *Ann.N.Y.Acad.Sci.Jour.* 125 (1966).802–806.

13  Schmale, A.H. & Iker, H.P.: "The affect of hopelessness and the
    development of cancer." *Jour.Psychosom.Med.* 28, 714–721 (1966).

14  Riley, V.: "Psychoendocrine influences on immunoreception and
    neoplasia." *Science* 212, 110–119 (1981).

15  Selye, H.: "Correlating stress and cancer." *Amer.Jour.Proct.Col.
    Rect.Surgery* Vol 30, 18–28 (1979).

16  Sklar, L.S. & Aisman, H.: "Stress and coping factors influence tumour
    growth." *Science* 205, 347–365 (1979).

17  Levenson: *Causes and Prevention of Cancer.*

18  LeShan, L.L. & Gassman, M.L.: "Some observations on psycho-

therapy with patients suffering from neoplastic disease." *Amer.Jour. Psychoth.* 12, 723–734 (1958).

19 Simonton, O.C., Matthews-Simonton, S. & Sparks, T.F.: "Psychological intervention in the treatment of cancer." *Psychosomatics* 21. 226–233 (1980).

20 Meares, A: "Vivid visualisation and dim visual awareness in the regression of cancer in meditation." *Jour.Amer.Soc.Psychosom. Dent.Med.* 25, 85–88 (1978).

21 Lansky, P.: "Possibility of hypnosis as an aid in cancer therapy." *Perspec.Biol.Med.* 25, 496–509 (1982).

22 Hedge, A.R.: "Hypnosis in cancer." *Brit.Jour.Med.Hypno.* 12, 2–5 (1960).

23 Meares, A.: "Stress, meditation and the regression of cancer." *Practitioner* 226, 1607–1609 (1982).

24 Cautela, J.R.: "Towards Pavlovian Theory of Cancer." *Scand.Jour. Behav.Therapy* 6, 117–142 (1977).

25 Dowling, S.J.: "Lourdes curees and their medical assessment" *Jour.Roy.Soc.Med* 77; 634–638.

26 Cunningham, A.J.: "Psychotherapy for Cancer" *Advances* 1[(4)]; 8–14 (1984).

27 Lerner: "Varieties of Integral Cancer Therapy." *Advances* (1985)

## Chapter 11

1 Melzac, R. & Wall, P.D.: "Pain Mechanisms: a New Theory." *Science* Vol 150, 1965, pg 971–979.

2 Moss, Dr Richard: *The I That is We* and *The Black Butterfly*. Open Gate Trust, 6 Goldney Rd, Clifton, Bristol.

3 LeShan, Lawrence: *You Can Fight for your Life*. Evans (USA).

4 Long, Haniel: *The Marvellous Adventure of Carbeza de Vaca*. Souvenir.

5 Illich, Ivan: *Deschooling Society*. Penguin.

6 *Jour.Complement.Med.Res.* Vol 1, no 1 Feb '86 onwards. RCCM.

# Glossary

**acute inflammatory reaction:**  Short or severe reaction of living tissue to injury, infection or irritation.

**adenocarcinoma:**  A malignant growth of glandular tissue.

**adriamycin:**  Anti-cancer drug.

**aetiology:**  A science dealing with the causation of disease.

**anaemia:**  Disorder of blood characterised by low number of red blood cells or haemoglobin.

**anaplastic:**  Having lost distinctive cell characteristics (indicative of very severe cancer).

**alpha brain wave:**  A type of brain wave measurable on electrical recording.

**ankylosing spondylosis:**  Disease of spinal column involving progressive joining together of back bones.

**anterior cervical fusion:**  Planned joining of backbones in the neck by surgery to prevent pain.

**anthroposophical:**  System of medicine described by Rudolf Steiner.

**anti-inflammatory drugs:**  Drugs to decrease pain, swelling and heat in sore joints or tissues.

**autogenic training:**  Profound relaxation technique.

**axillary lymph nodes:**  Lymph nodes in armpit.

**axillary lymph node clearance:**  Surgical removal of lymph nodes in armpit.

**axillary tail (of left breast):**  Part of breast nearest to armpit.

**BACUP:**  A cancer support network.

**barium enema:**  Insertion of radio-opaque barium into anus, rectum and colon with subsequent x-ray to look for the presence of cancer.

**benign:**  Innocent (opposite of malignant).

**biofeedback:**  Use of the body's signals.
(e.g. electrical skin resistance, heartbeat, breathing rate) to assess state of stress and measure effectiveness of relaxation techniques.

**biofeedback meter:**  Meter to measure electrical skin resistance.

**biopsy:**  Removal and examination (usually microscopic) of tissue or other material from the living body for purpose of diagnosis.

**bronchoscopy:**  Direct visualisation of inside of bronchus.

**bronchus:**  Tubes leading from the windpipe into the lungs.

**BUPA hospital:**  Private hospital.

**C3/4:**  Space between third and fourth neck bones.

**C4/5:**  Space between fourth and fifth neck bones.

**carcinogenic:**  Producing cancer.

**carcinogens:**  Any cancer producing substance.

**carcinomatous:**  Pertaining to or the nature of cancer.

**catecholamines:**  Nerve transmitter substances released in excitement and stress, e.g. adrenaline.

**catharsis:**   A cleansing, outpouring of emotion.

**catheter:**   Tube inserted into bladder for automatic drainage of urine.

**CAT Scan:**   Co-axial Tomagraphic Scan (sophisticated internal body diagnostic image).

**chemotherapy:**   The treatment of disease by chemical agents.

**chiropractor:**   Person who treats disease by the manipulation of the spinal column and joints.

**clinically clear:**   Absence of detectable cancer in the body.

**clinical signs:**   Evidence of disease found by doctors on examining patients.

**co-factors:**   Chemical substances occuring naturally with and enhancing chemical activity of other chemical substances, e.g. vitamins.

**colonic:**   Relating to colon, last part of the large intestine.

**colostomy:**   Cutting surgically and bringing of the colon to the skin, thereby creating an artificial anus on the wall of the abdomen.

**coronary heart disease:**   Narrowing of the artery supplying heart muscle.

**coronary thrombosis:**   Blockage of the artery supplying heart muscle.

**corpuscle:**   Blood cell.

**cortisone:**   A hormone secreted by adrenal gland.

**cranial osteopathy:**   Balancing of the body's energy by gentle manipulation of the flow of the cerebrospinal fluid.

**cyst:**   A sac containing fluid or semi-solid material.

**cyclophosphamide:**   Anti-cancer drug.

**cystoscope:**   Instrument for direct visualisation of the bladder.

**cystoscopy:**   Direct visualisation of the bladder.

**dermal infiltration:**   Growth of cancer cells into the skin.

**drips:**   Drop by drop infusion of fluid into a vein.

**ductal carcinoma:**   Cancer of milk duct in breast.

**duodenum:**   First part of small intestine.

**dyslexia:**   Impairment of reading ability.

**emphysema:**   Destruction of lung tissue structure.

**endocrine:**   Gland secreting into tissue or bloodstream.

**endorphins:**   Morphine like nerve transmitter substances.

**enzymes:**   Chemicals which break down foods into absorbable molecules.

**epigastrium:**   Upper middle region of the abdomen.

**epithelia:**   Membranes covering internal and external structures of the body.

**Ewing's disease:**   Cancer of bone.

**fungating:**   Rapid growth of tumour breaking the surface of the skin.

**gastro-intestinal:**   Pertaining to stomach or intestine.

**haemorrhage:**   Severe bleeding.

**hemicolectomy:**   Removal of approximately half the colon.

**hernia:** Abnormal protrusion of a body organ through an abnormal weakness or opening in the body wall.

**Hippocratic Oath:** Oath taken by doctors on qualifying.

**histology:** Microscopic study of tissues.

**Hodgkin's disease:** Cancer of the lymphatic system.

**holistic:** Relating to the whole person, the whole being greater than the sum of the parts.

**homoeopathic:** System of medicine involving the treatment of symptoms with minute doses of substances which produce like symptoms in the well.

**houseman:** Most junior hospital doctor.

**hypothalamus:** Region of the brain controlling the hormone system of the body.

**hypothesized:** Supposition assumed as a basis of reasoning.

**hysterectomy:** Removal of the womb.

**immune system:** Cells and organs of the body which defend it against invasion or disease.

**infiltrative cells:** Cancer cells which are growing into surrounding tissue.

**inoperable:** Not suitable to be operated upon (ref. cancer; too widely spread to be removable).

**intervertebral discs:** Cartilage discs between vertebrae (backbones).

**intravenously:** Within or into a vein.

**iridology:** Study of the iris of the eye for diagnostic purposes.

**irritable bowel syndrome:** Inflammation of the bowel resulting in impaired functioning (pain, diarrhoea and constipation).

**Iscador:** Anti-cancer treatment made from mistletoe.

**ischaemic heart disease:** see Coronary heart disease.

**language centre:** Part of brain in which speech is formed.

**laparotomy:** Incision of abdominal wall.

**lesion:** Pathological change in a bodily tissue.

**leukaemia:** Cancer of white blood cells.

**limbic system:** Part of brain involved in emotions.

**local recurrence:** Recurrence of cancer at site of previous removal.

**lumpectomy:** Removal of cancerous breast lump (rather than the whole breast).

**lymph:** Fluid flowing in lymph vessels collected from tissues and returned into the large veins.

**lymph nodes:** Collection of protective cells found at intervals along the lymph vessels.

**lymphoedema:** Swelling which occurs in the tissues when lymph flow is blocked.

**malignant:** Virulent and dangerous. That which is likely to have a fatal termination.

**mammograph:** X-ray of the breast.

**mandible:** Jawbone.

**mantra:** Eastern chant.

**mastectomy:** Removal of a breast.

**mediastinal:** Within the space between the lungs.

**mediastinoscopy:** Visualisation of the space between the lungs.

**mega-dose:** Extremely large dose.

**melanoma:** Cancer of the pigment-producing cells of the skin.

**menopause:** Cessation of menstruation.

**metabolic:** Pertaining to the series of chemical changes in the living body by which life is maintained.

**metabolic treatment:** Treatment with basic body chemicals eg. vitamins and minerals.

**metastasis:** Growth of cancer in a new and sometimes distant site.

**mineral:** Non-organic substance occuring in the earth (some of which are vital for life).

**multi-factorial:** Having many causes.

**myeloma:** A primary, malignant tumour of bone marrow.

**necrotic:** Dead tissue.

**necrotic calcified material:** Dead tissue which has become chalky.

**neuro-endocrine:** Relating to the nervous and glandular systems.

**neurological:** Relating to the nervous system.

**oncologist:** Cancer specialist.

**oncology:** Study of cancer.

**orthodox treatment:** Standard medical treatment offered by doctors and hospitals.

**orthopaedic:** Branch of surgery relating to the skeleton.

**palpable:** Able to be felt.

**palpitations:** Abnormally rapid or irregular heartbeat.

**pancreas:** Abdominal organ secreting insulin and enzymes of digestion.

**parasympathetic nervous system:** Automatic section of the nervous system regulating 'internal house-keeping' functions of the body.

**paratracheal:** Next to the windpipe.

**Patey mastectomy:** Mastectomy pioneered by Patey.

**pathological:** Study of cause and nature of disease.

**pharmacological:** Relating to drugs.

**physiological:** Pertaining to the normal function of the body.

**pituitary:** Central gland in the brain controlling all other glands in the body.

**placebo effect:** Beneficial effect of the giving of treatment which is not due to the treatment's inherent efficacy.

**plasmacytoma:** Tumour of plasma cells.

**poorly differentiated adenocarcinoma:** Very severe adenocarcinoma.

**pre-cursor:** Chemical building block or fore-runner.

**primary:**   Tissue of origin of cancer.

**prognosis:**   Forecast of the probable result of a disease.

**prospective trial:**   Scientific research using no old data.

**prosthesis:**   Artificial substitute for a missing part.

**psychoneuroimmunology:**   Science of the mutual influence of the mind, glandular and immune systems.

**psychosomatic:**   Illness where emotional factors produce physical symptoms.

**radical operation:**   Uncompromised, drastic removal of cancer and all surrounding tissue.

**radiographer:**   Person who takes x-rays.

**radiotherapy:**   Treatment of cancer with radiation.

**reflexology:**   Diagnosis and treatment of disease through foot massage.

**remission:**   Period of abatement of a disease.

**resection:**   Excision of a considerable portion of a structure.

**respiratory:**   Relating to breathing or incorporation of oxygen into the tissues.

**right brain function/activity:**   Brain activity associated with creativity, intuition etc.

**rodent ulcer:**   Skin cancer.

**screening tests:**   Tests performed in the absence of symptons to look for the presence of disease.

**secondaries:**   Cancer appearing in sites other than organ of origin, e.g. breast cancer appearing in the lungs.

**septicaemia:**   Infection of the blood.

**signs:**   See Clinical signs.

**squamous cell carcinoma:**   Cancer arising in covering membranes of the body.

**steroid:**   Group of naturally occuring chemicals including sex hormones, cortisone, bile acids etc.

**steroid secretion:**   Production of steroids by the body (in response to stress in this instance).

**steroid therapy:**   Administration of synthetic steroids to suppress the functioning of the immune system and thereby decrease inflammation and swelling.

**superior vena cava:**   Vein returning blood from the upper part of the body to the heart.

**sympathetic nervous system:**   Automatic section of the nervous system involved in reaction to outside threat.

**tamoxifen:**   Drug blocking the effect of oestrogen (which is thought to cause some breast cancers to grow).

**TB:** Tuberculosis. Infection of the organs of the body with Mycobacterium Tuberculosis.

**thoracotomy:**   Operation involving the opening of the chest.

**thyroid:**   Gland in the neck controlling metabolic rate.

**thyrotoxicosis:**   Disease state resulting from overactive thyroid gland.

**toxins:**   Poisons.

**transverse colon:**   Portion of large intestine which crosses the upper part of the abdomen.

**tumour:**   A mass of abnormal tissue which grows at the body's expense.

**ultrasound:**   Diagnostic imaging technique using sound waves.

**valium:**   Sedative, anxiety reducing medication.

**vascular surgeon:**   Surgeon specialising in blood vessels.

**vincristine:**   Anti-cancer drug.

**vertebrae:**   Backbones.

**vertebral venous fistula:**   Abnormal connection between veins and arteries in the neck region.

**vitamin:**   Chemicals which are essential for normal body functioning which cannot be synthesized by the body.

**white cells:**   Blood cells involved in defence of the body.

**white corpuscles:**   See white cells.

# Bibliography

Brohn, Penny: *The Bristol Programme*. Century.
Rippon, Saddhya: *The Bristol Recipe Book*. Century.
Clyne, Rachel: *Coping with Cancer*. Thorsons.
Gawain, Shakti: *Creative Visualisation*. Bantam.
Hyne-Jones, T.W.: *Dictionary of Bach Flower Remedies*. Daniel.
Chaitow, Leon: *End to Cancer*. Thorsons.
Howard, Alex: *Finding a Way*. Gateway.
Brohn, Penny: *Gentle Giants*. Century.
Jampolsky, J.J.: *Goodbye to Guilt*. Bantam.
Levine, Stephen: *Healing into Life and Death*. Gateway.
Bach, Edward: *Heal Thyself*. Daniel.
LeShan, Lawrence: *Holistic Health*. Turnstone.
LeShan, Lawrence: *How to Meditate*. Turnstone.
Jampolsky, J.J.: *Love is Letting Go of Fear*. Celestial Arts (USA).
Siegel, Dr Bernie: *Love, Medicine and Miracles*. Rider.
Weiner, Michael: *Maximum Immunity*. Gateway.
Harrison, Shirley: *New Approaches to Cancer*. Century.
Gear, Alan: *Organic Food Guide*. Dent.
Bennett, Dr Glin: *Patients and Their Doctors*. Bailliere Tindall.
Bennett, Dr Glin: *The Wound and the Doctor*. Bailliere Tindall.
Kenton, Leslie & Susanne: *Raw Energy*. Arrow.
Kenton, Leslie: *Raw Energy Recipes*. Arrow.
Weeks, Dr Claire: *Self Help for your Nerves*. Angus and Robertson.
Madders, Jane: *Stress and Relaxation*. Macdonald.
Meares, Dr Ainslie: *The Wealth Within*. Ashgrove.
Ferrucci, Piero: *What We May Be*. Turnstone.
Gawler, Ian: *You Can Conquer Cancer*. Hill of Content (Aust).
LeShan, Lawrence: *You Can Fight for your Life*. Turnstone Press.
Rainwater, Janette: *You're in Charge*. Turnstone.

# Tapes

Manning, Matthew: Breathe.
            *Cancer: A Positive Approach for Men.*
            *Cancer: A Positive approach for Women.*
            *Release from Phobias.*
Brohn, Penny: *Helping with Healing.*
            *Introduction to the Cancer Help Centre.*
Greatorex, Chistopher: *First Steps in Meditation.*
Pietroni, Dr Patrick: *Introduction to Meditation.*
LeShan, Lawrence: *Mobilising Inner Resources of Self-Healing.*
Adams, Jenni: *Relax and Unwind.*
How, Ludi & Brookman, Michael: *Relaxation and Meditation.*

Many of these books and all of these tapes are available directly from **The Cancer Help Centre, Grove House, Clifton, Bristol, BS8 4PG.**

Some other GATEWAY BOOKS that might interest you:

**Finding a Way**: *A Realist's Introduction to Self-Help Therapy*
by Alex Howard
"This exceptionally helpful and down-to-earth book is a revealing, teach yourself course in removing those masks we hide behind, in getting to know ourselves and others better...providing many practical guidelines of who we really are and how much we can truly give to each other. I strongly recommend this valuable book". *Science of Thought Review*
224pp            paper            £5.95            (US $11.95)

**The Magic of Mind Power**: *Awareness Techniques for the Creative Mind*
by Duncan McColl
This is a practical guide to the immense potential of the unconscious mind. It explains how and why visualisation, creative imagery and self-hypnosis work; areas now commonly used in the healing professions. This self-help guide tackles questions such as Can I learn from my dreams? How do subliminal tapes work?, and provides techniques which help to eliminate negative conditioning which can lead to bad health, lack of energy and low self-confidence.
192pp            Illus.            paper            £5.95            (US $10.95)

**A Rose to a Sick Friend**: *A Positive Way to Approach Your Illness*
by Tessa Goldhawk
This book offers a new way of coping with illness, pain, stress and worry. Written in a light style and interspersed with cartoons, jokes and exercises, it is nonetheless serious in purpose, the underlying message being that to some extent we create our own illnesses, and an understanding of this is the key to recovery. You are taken through a six-stage process, including accepting illness, learning from it, and learning to throw it off.
192pp            Illus.            paper            £5.95            (US $10.95)

**Reducing the Risk of Alzheimer's**
by Michael Weiner PhD
An important background book on the degenerative disease that affects 1 in 8 of the population. Recent research has shown the connection between aluminum deposits in the brain and Alzheimer's, which is of great concern as aluminum is now a very common constituent in food preparation. The book includes a detailed program of preventative action for those in the early stages of the disease, and will give hope to many.
176pp            paper            £5.95            (US $10.95)

**Who Dies?**: *An Investigation of Conscious Living and Conscious Dying*
by Stephen Levine
How to participate fully in life as the perfect preparation for whatever comes next, be it sorrow or joy, loss or gain, death, or a new wonderment at life.
332pp            paper            £7.95            (not USA)